WITHDRAWN

Workbook for Diagnostic Medical Sonography

A GUIDE TO CLINICAL PRACTICE, THE VASCULAR SYSTEM

D1591372

WITHDRAWN

Workbook for Diagnostic Medical Sonography

A GUIDE TO CLINICAL PRACTICE, THE VASCULAR SYSTEM

Nathalie Garbani, EdD, RVT
Assistant Professor
Nova Southeastern University
Fort Lauderdale, Florida

Rachel Kendoll, MEd, RVT
Program Director, Vascular Technology
Spokane Community College
Spokane, Washington

Wolters Kluwer | Lippincott Williams & Wilkins
Health
Philadelphia • Baltimore • New York • London
Buenos Aires • Hong Kong • Sydney • Tokyo

Publisher: Julie K. Stegman
Senior Product Manager: Heather Rybacki
Product Manager: Kristin Royer
Marketing Manager: Shauna Kelley
Design Coordinator: Joan Wendt
Art Director: Jennifer Clements
Manufacturing Coordinator: Margie Orzech
Production Services: Absolute Service, Inc.

Copyright © 2013 by Lippincott Williams & Wilkins, a Wolters Kluwer business

351 West Camden Street   Two Commerce Square
Baltimore, MD 21201   2001 Market Street
                                          Philadelphia, PA 19103

First Edition

All rights reserved. This book is protected by copyright. No part of it may be reproduced in any form by any means, including photocopying, or utilized by any information storage and retrieval system without written permission from the copyright owner, except for brief quotations embodied in critical articles and reviews. Materials appearing in the book prepared by individuals as part of their official duties as U.S. government employees are not covered by the above-mentioned copyright.

Printed in China.

Library of Congress Cataloging-in-Publication Data
Cataloging-in-Publication Data available upon request.

Care has been taken to confirm the accuracy of the information presented and to describe generally accepted practices. However, the authors, editors, and publisher are not responsible for errors or omissions or for any consequences from application of the information in this book and make no warranty, express or implied, with respect to the contents of the publication. Application of the information in a particular situation remains the professional responsibility of the practitioner.

The authors, editors, and publisher have exerted every effort to ensure that drug selection and dosage set forth in this text are in accordance with current recommendations and practice at the time of publication. However, in view of ongoing research, changes in government regulations, and the constant flow of information relating to drug therapy and drug reactions, the reader is urged to check the package insert for each drug for any change in indications and dosage and for added warnings and precautions. This is particularly important when the recommended agent is a new or infrequently employed drug.

Some drugs and medical devices presented in this publication have Food and Drug Administration (FDA) clearance for limited use in restricted research settings. It is the responsibility of the health care provider to ascertain the FDA status of each drug or device planned for use in their clinical practice.

To purchase additional copies of this book, call our customer service department at **(800) 638-3030** or fax orders to **(301) 223-2320**. International customers should call **(301) 223-2300**.
Visit Lippincott Williams & Wilkins on the Internet: **http://www.lww.com.** Lippincott Williams & Wilkins customer service representatives are available from 8:30 am to 6:00 pm, EST.

10 9 8 7 6 5 4 3 2 1

Contents

PART 6 • MISCELLANEOUS

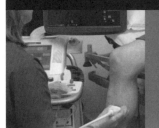

1 Vascular Anatomy

REVIEW OF GLOSSARY TERMS

MATCHING

Match the key terms with their definitions.

Key Terms

1. _____ Artery

2. _____ Arteriole

3. _____ Capillary

4. _____ Venule

5. _____ Vein

Definitions

a. A small blood vessel with only endothelium and basement membrane through which exchange of nutrients and waste occurs

b. A small vein that is continuous with a capillary

c. A blood vessel that carries blood away from the heart

d. A small artery with a muscular wall; a terminal artery, which continues into the capillary network

e. A blood vessel that carries blood toward the heart

ANATOMY AND PHYSIOLOGY REVIEW

IMAGE LABELING

Complete the labels in the images that follow.

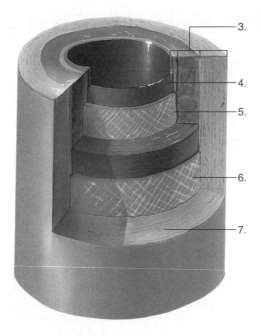

3.

4.

5.

6.

7.

1. _____

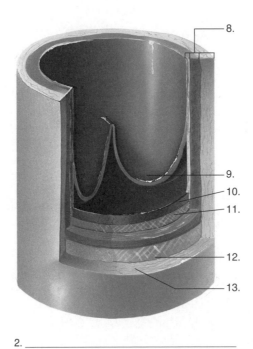

8.

9.

10.

11.

12.

13.

2. _____

Schematic diagram of arterial and venous walls.

CHAPTER REVIEW

MULTIPLE CHOICE

1. Exchange of oxygen, carbon dioxide, waste, and nutrients occur at which level of the circulatory system?
   a. Aorta
   b. Inferior vena cava
   c. Arterioles
   d. Capillaries

2. Which of the following statements regarding the exchange at the level of the capillaries is FALSE?
   a. Nutrients and oxygen exchange occurs at the arterial side
   b. Nutrients and oxygen exchange is simultaneous to carbon dioxide and waste exchange
   c. Nutrients and oxygen exchange occurs at the venous side
   d. Exchange occurs at the venous and arterial side

3. Capillary permeability to large molecules is:
   a. The same in all tissues
   b. Different and characteristics to every tissues
   c. Selective only in the brain
   d. Selective only in the liver

4. Why can arterioles control the resistance of the vascular bed?
   a. They have concentric layers of smooth muscle cells
   b. They are the smallest arteries in the circulatory system
   c. They are the vessels leading to the capillaries
   d. They have all three main layers of tissue (intima, media, and adventitia)

5. Which of the following is NOT an example of a large muscular artery?
   a. The common carotid arteries
   b. The common femoral arteries
   c. The common iliac arteries
   d. The aorta

6. The main difference between arteries and veins of a similar size resides in the composition of the:
   a. Tunica media
   b. Adventitia
   c. Tunica intima
   d. Endothelium

7. Which of the following is NOT an example of a large vein?
   a. The portal vein
   b. The inferior vena cava
   c. The superior vena cava
   d. The jugular vein

8. Which of the following statements on venous valves is FALSE?
   a. They allow for bidirectional flow under normal conditions
   b. They are more numerous in the veins of the lower extremities
   c. They are usually absent from veins in the thorax and abdomen
   d. They have only two leaflets

9. Valves are formed by which of the following structures from the blood vessel?
   a. Two semilunar cusps
   b. The elastic and collagen fibers from the basement membrane
   c. Projections of the intima layer
   d. Projections of the media layer

10. Which of the following statements regarding the first branch of the internal carotid artery is FALSE?
    a. The ophthalmic artery is usually the first branch at the petrous level
    b. The ophthalmic artery is usually the first branch at the cavernous level
    c. The ophthalmic artery is usually the first branch at the cerebral level
    d. The internal carotid artery does not have branches

11. Where does the left common carotid artery typically arise from?
    a. The left subclavian artery
    b. The aortic arch
    c. The innominate artery
    d. The right subclavian artery

12. Which of the following statements regarding the venous drainage of the head and neck is FALSE?
    a. Drainage occurs in the posterior portion via vertebral veins
    b. Vertebral veins are formed by a dense venous plexus
    c. The external jugular veins drain into the innominate veins
    d. The internal jugular veins drain into the innominate veins

13. Which tissues do branches of the right or left subclavian arteries supply?
    a. The brain and neck
    b. The thoracic wall and shoulder
    c. The aortic arch
    d. Both A and B

14. Which of the following arteries is NOT typically a branch of the ulnar arteries?
    a. The radial artery
    b. The interosseous artery
    c. The recurrent ulnar artery
    d. The superficial palmar arch

15. Which of the following is NOT a superficial vein of the upper extremities?
    a. The interosseus veins
    b. The basilic veins
    c. The cephalic veins
    d. The medial antebrachial veins

16. What are the three branches of the celiac trunk or celiac artery?
    a. The SMA, IMA, and hepatic artery
    b. The SMA, right, and left gastric artery
    c. The splenic, left gastric, and hepatic arteries
    d. The splenic, right gastric, and hepatic arteries

17. What are the internal iliac arteries also known as?
    a. The hypergastric arteries
    b. The hypogastric arteries
    c. The epigastric arteries
    d. The subgastric arteries

18. Which of the following are branches of the popliteal arteries?
    a. The tibial and peroneal arteries
    b. The genicular and sural arteries
    c. The anterior and posterior tibial arteries
    d. The anterior tibial artery and tibioperoneal trunk

19. Where does the deep venous system of the lower extremities start?
    a. The deep plantar arch
    b. The medial plantar arch
    c. The lateral plantar arch
    d. The dorsal venous arch

20. Typically, what happens as the popliteal vein and artery passes through the adductor canal?
    a. The vein moves from medial to lateral of the artery
    b. The vein moves from lateral to medial of the artery
    c. The vein moves from anterior to posterior of the artery
    d. The vein moves from posterior to anterior of the artery

FILL-IN-THE-BLANK

1. Exchange of gasses, nutrients, and wastes can only occur at the level of _____ in the circulatory system.

2. The venous side of the capillaries is drained by _____.

3. Arterioles have been called the _____ of the circulatory system.

4. Arterioles are the main control of _____ of the circulatory system.

5. Arteries are classified not only according to size but also in the composition of the _____.

6. The femoral arteries, the brachial arteries, and the mesenteric arteries are examples of _____.

7. Lower extremities veins have _____ walls than upper extremities veins.

8. The thickest layer in large veins is _____.

9. The adventitia in large veins contains _____.

10. The valves found in veins are called

_____ because they have two

semilunar leaflets.

11. The petrous, cavernous, and cerebral levels

correspond to the _____ portion

of the internal carotid artery.

12. A unique arrangement of the intracranial branches

of the internal carotid and vertebral arteries

serving as an important collateral network is called

_____.

13. The first and largest branch of the aortic arch is the

_____.

14. Typically, the _____ is considered

the first and largest branch of the brachial artery.

15. The upper extremity superficial vein coursing along

the medial border of the biceps muscle is the

_____.

16. The bronchial, esophageal, phrenic, intercostal,

and subcostal arteries are branches of the

_____.

17. The right and left common iliac arteries bifurcate

from the abdominal aorta, typically at the level of the

_____.

18. The other name of the deep femoral artery is

_____.

19. The continuation of the lateral segment of the dorsal

venous arch is _____.

20. The veins that pass between the tibia and fibula

through the upper part of the interosseous membrane

are the _____.

SHORT ANSWER

1. Why have arterioles been called the stopcocks of the circulatory system?

2. Why are arterioles able to be the main control of resistance in the vascular system?

3. Arteries, veins, arterioles, and venules have three basic cellular layers known as what?

4. The liver has a unique arrangement of vessels and receives blood from what two sources?

5. In 96% of individuals, the venous drainage of the liver is through what?

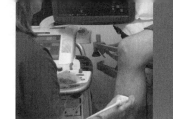

2 Arterial Physiology

REVIEW OF GLOSSARY TERMS

MATCHING

Match the key terms with their definitions.

Key Terms

1. _____ Potential energy

2. _____ Kinetic energy

3. _____ Poiseuille's law

4. _____ Laminar flow

5. _____ Viscosity

6. _____ Inertia

Definitions

a. The energy of work or motion; in the vascular system, it is in part represented by the velocity of blood flow

b. The stored or resting energy; in the vascular system, it is the intravascular pressure

c. Flow of a liquid in which it travels smoothly in parallel layers

d. The law that states the volume flow of a liquid flowing through a vessel is directly proportional to the pressure of the liquid and the fourth power of the radius and is inversely proportional to the viscosity of the liquid and the length of the vessel

e. The tendency of a body at rest to stay at rest or a body in motion to stay in motion

f. The property of a fluid that resists the force tending to cause fluid to flow

CHAPTER REVIEW

MULTIPLE CHOICE

1. Where in the vascular system is the lowest energy represented by the lowest pressure located?
   a. The right atrium
   b. The left atrium
   c. The right ventricle
   d. The left ventricle

2. Which of the following statements regarding the gravitational energy and hydrostatic pressure is FALSE?
   a. They are components of the total energy in the vascular system
   b. They tend to cancel each other
   c. They are components of the kinetic energy in the vascular system
   d. They are expressed in relation to a reference point

3. What can blood flow also be referred to as?
   a. Velocity
   b. Volume flow
   c. Displacement with respect to time
   d. Expressed in cm/s

4. In the entire vascular system, the cross-sectional area of vessels:
   a. Increases from the aorta to the capillary level
   b. Decreases from the aorta to the capillary level
   c. Remains the same from the aorta to the capillary level
   d. Increases only at the level of the arterioles

5. Which of the following statements regarding the velocity of the blood flow is FALSE?
   a. Velocity refers to the rate of displacement of blood in time
   b. The velocity of the blood increases from the capillaries to the venous system
   c. The velocity of the blood increases from the aorta to the capillaries
   d. The velocity of the blood changes with cross-sectional area of the vessels

6. Which of the following could NOT be used as a unit to measure flow volume?
   a. ml/s
   b. m/s
   c. cl/min
   d. l/min

7. In the vascular system, what represents the potential difference or voltage in Ohm's law?
   a. The volume flow
   b. The resistance
   c. The pressure gradient
   d. The radius

8. Changes in resistance in the vascular system will be significantly affected by which of the following?
   a. Changes in the volume flow
   b. Changes in the velocity
   c. Changes in the viscosity of the blood
   d. Changes in the radius of vessels

9. Which of the following will arrangements of elements in parallel in a system allow for?
   a. Lower total resistance than when elements are in series
   b. Higher total resistance then when elements are in series
   c. Does not affect the total resistance of a system
   d. Disrupting flow in collaterals

10. Which of the following characterizes low-resistance flow?
    a. Retrograde flow
    b. Alternating antegrade/retrograde flow
    c. Antegrade flow
    d. Constriction of arteriolar bed

11. Which of the following about high-resistance flow characteristics is FALSE?
    a. The flow profile may be two to three phases
    b. The flow displays alternating antegrade/retrograde flow
    c. The flow profile is due to vasoconstriction of arterioles
    d. The flow profile is due to vasodilatation of arterioles

12. What is the flow profile referred to as at the entrance of a vessel?
    a. Plug flow
    b. Laminar flow
    c. Turbulent flow
    d. Streamlined flow

13. Which of the following statements regarding laminar flow is FALSE?
    a. The layers of cells at the center of the vessels move the fastest
    b. The layers of cells at the wall of the vessels do not move
    c. The velocity at the center of the vessels is half the mean velocity
    d. The difference in velocities between layers is due to friction

14. What is required to move blood flow in a turbulent system?
    a. Higher velocities
    b. Greater pressure
    c. Larger radius
    d. Smaller radius

15. What is the function of the hydraulic filter of the arterial system (composed of the elastic arteries and high-resistance arterioles)?
    a. Ensure adequate gas/nutrient exchange in the arteries
    b. Convert the cardiac output flow to steady flow
    c. Ensure adequate conduction of the pressure wave
    d. Distribute flow to the capillaries

16. In diastole, what is the conversion of potential energy into blood flow due to?
    a. Ejection of the stroke volume from the heart
    b. The elastic recoil of the arteries
    c. The cardiac contraction
    d. The hydraulic filter

17. What is the resistance in the arterial system controlled by?
    a. The contraction and relaxation of smooth muscle cells in the media of arterioles
    b. The contraction and relaxation of the heart
    c. The contraction and relaxation of muscle cells in the surrounding tissue
    d. The capacitance of the arterial system

18. Which of the following will norepinephrine released by the sympathetic nervous system do?
    a. Trigger the relaxation of smooth muscle cells in arterioles
    b. Trigger the contraction of smooth muscle cells in arterioles
    c. Not have any effect on the smooth muscle cells in arterioles
    d. Not have any effect on the tone of the arteriole walls

19. Most prominently, abnormal energy losses in the arterial system would result from pathologies such as obstruction and/or stenoses because of which of the following?
    a. The increased length of the stenosis
    b. The friction from the atherosclerotic plaque
    c. The decreased in the vessel's radius
    d. The increased viscosity

20. Which of the following statements about collateral vessels is FALSE?
    a. Collaterals appear *de novo*
    b. The resistance in collaterals is mostly fixed
    c. Vasodilator drugs have little effect on collaterals
    d. Midzone collaterals are small intramuscular branches

FILL-IN-THE-BLANK

1. In the human body, the major component of the blood influencing viscosity is _____.

2. The highest pressure in the vascular system (of approximately 120 mm Hg) is found in the

   _____.

3. The farther from the reference point in the right atrium, the _____ the hydrostatic pressure.

4. The principle stating that the total energy remains constant from one point to another without changes in flow velocity is the _____.

5. Inertia and viscosity are two components of the vascular system contributing to

   _____.

6. In the vascular system, if the volume of blood or flow remains the same, an increase in flow velocity should trigger a _____ in the area of the vessels.

7. The law defined by the statement that the current through two points is directly proportional to the potential difference across the two points and inversely proportional to the resistance between them is _____.

8. The total resistance in a system where the elements are arranged in series is _____.

9. A low-resistance flow profile characteristically displays _____ flow throughout the cardiac cycle.

10. The third phase seen in high-resistance flow profile is related to _____ of the proximal vessels.

11. After exercise and under normal conditions, the resistance of the tissues in the lower extremities will change from _____.

12. In laminar flow, the "layers" of cells at the center of the vessel move _____ than the layers closest to the wall of the vessel.

13. Turbulence in a blood vessel is mostly the result of change of velocity and _____.

14. The Reynolds number above which turbulence of flow starts to occur is _____.

15. The arterial system can be compared to _____ of the resistance/capacitance filters of an electrical circuit.

16. Pulse pressure in the arterial system is the difference between _____ pressure.

17. A drop in interstitial _____ will trigger the arterioles to dilate.

18. At the entrance and exit of a stenosis, there will be energy _____.

19. Energy losses due to stenosis will be more pronounced with less diameter reduction in a _____ resistance system.

20. Under normal conditions, blood flow _____ by at least three to five times the resting value.

SHORT ANSWER

1. In the human circulatory system, the total energy of the system is a balance between what?

2. Hematocrit represents what?

3. In the human circulatory system, when does inertial loss occur?

4. What causes blood in the vascular system, as any other fluid in a closed system, to move from one point to the next?

5. Why does the velocity of the blood decrease as the blood travels from the aorta to the arterioles?

6. Reynolds number is used to express turbulence in the vascular system. This number is directly proportional to what? And indirectly proportional to what?

IMAGE EVALUATION/PATHOLOGY

From this Doppler spectrum, you could conclude that:
1. The vessel sampled was:

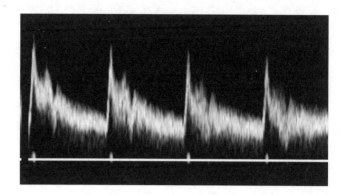

2. The vessel sampled supplies:

3. The velocities for this vessel are:

4. The Doppler spectrum suggests:

From this Doppler spectrum, you could conclude that:
5. The vessel sampled was:

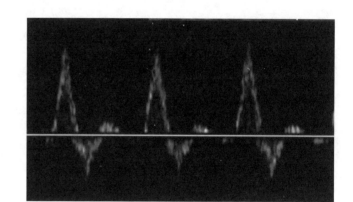

6. The vessel sampled supplies:

7. The velocities for this vessel are:

8. The Doppler spectrum suggests: pathology-no
pathology-cannot tell

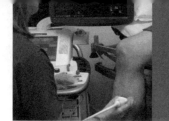

3 Venous Physiology

REVIEW OF GLOSSARY TERMS

MATCHING

Match the key terms with their definitions.

Key Terms

1. _____ Hydrostatic pressure

2. _____ Transmural pressure

3. _____ Edema

4. _____ Venous insufficiency

Definitions

a. The pressure exerted on the walls of a vessel
b. Excessive accumulation of fluid in cells, tissues, or cavities of the body
c. The pressure within the vascular system due to the weight of a column of blood
d. Abnormal retrograde flow in veins

ANATOMY AND PHYSIOLOGY REVIEW

IMAGE LABELING

Complete the labels in the images that follow.

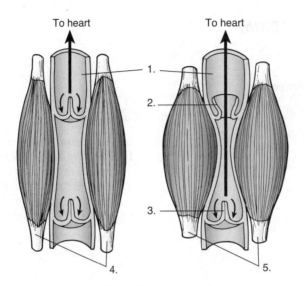

Structure of a venous valve.

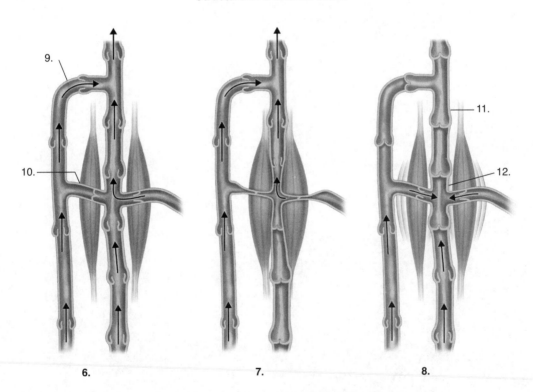

Patterns of normal venous flow at rest and with calf contraction.

CHAPTER REVIEW

MULTIPLE CHOICE

1. Approximately how much blood does the venous portion of the vascular system hold?
   a. 66% to 67% of the total volume of blood
   b. One-third of the total volume of blood
   c. 3% to 4% of the total volume of blood
   d. Half of the total volume of blood

2. Which of the following statements about the resistance of the venous system is NOT correct?
   a. Veins offer resistance to flow through increase in pressure
   b. Veins offer natural resistance to flow in some areas of the body
   b. An elliptical shape in the vein increases the resistance
   d. A circular shape in the vein decreases the resistance

3. Which of the following veins do NOT offer natural resistance to flow in the venous system?
   a. The subclavian veins
   b. The innominate veins
   c. The jugular veins
   d. The inferior vena cava

4. In a 6-foot-tall individual in a standing position, the hydrostatic pressure will add approximately how much?
   a. 170 mm Hg of pressure at the ankle
   b. 100 mm Hg of pressure at the ankle
   c. 15 mm Hg of pressure at the ankle
   d. 20 mm Hg of pressure at the ankle

5. Veins would collapse if the intravascular pressure in that vessel drops to what level?
   a. Below -50 mm Hg
   b. Below -5 mm Hg
   c. Below 5 mm Hg
   d. Below 20 mm Hg

6. What pressure gradient would the hydrostatic pressure in an arm lifted above the head provide?
   a. 100 mm Hg
   b. 80 mm Hg
   c. 40 mm Hg
   d. 20 mm Hg

7. Once a vein has acquired a circular shape, the volume of blood in the vessel can only change with which of the following?
   a. Large increase of pressure
   b. Little increase of pressure
   c. No increase of pressure
   d. Negative pressure

8. When an individual moves from a supine to a standing position, which of the following pressures specific to the venous system increases?
   a. The osmotic pressure
   b. The hydrostatic pressure
   c. The transmural pressure
   d. The gravitational force

9. Which of the following is NOT a force influencing the movement of fluid at the level of the capillaries (in or out of the surrounding tissue)?
   a. Intracapillary pressure
   b. Interstitial osmotic pressure
   c. Capillary osmotic pressure
   d. Transmural pressure

10. The role of the action of calf muscles (aka calf muscle pump) under normal circumstances is to offset fluid loss in interstitial tissue because of what reason?
    a. It helps increase the venous pressure
    b. It helps decrease the venous pressure
    c. It helps decrease the osmotic pressure
    d. It helps decrease the interstitial pressure

11. Under normal circumstances, the inspiration phase of respiration results in all of the following except:
    a. An ascent of the diaphragm
    b. A descent of the diaphragm
    c. An increase in intra-abdominal pressure
    d. A decrease in intrathoracic pressure

12. With total or partial thrombosis of major veins of the lower extremities, it is not unusual for the flow profile from proximal nonoccluded veins from the lower extremities to do what?
    a. Change from continuous to phasic
    b. Change from phasic to pulsatile
    c. Change from pulsatile to phasic
    d. Change from phasic to continuous

13. Which of the following is essential to ensure the proper functioning of the calf muscle pump under normal conditions when an individual is standing or sitting?
    a. Properly functioning valves
    b. Well-developed gastrocnemius muscle venous sinusoids
    c. Well-developed soleal muscle venous sinusoids
    d. A superficial venous system

14. Contraction of an efficient calf muscle pump under normal conditions can generate a pressure of how much?
    a. At least 50 mm Hg
    b. At least 15 mm Hg
    c. At least 200 mm Hg
    d. At least 5 mm Hg

15. Primary and secondary varicose veins are distinguishable mainly because primary varicose veins:
    a. Do not affect the small saphenous vein
    b. Develop in the absence of deep venous thrombosis
    c. Do not rely on the calf muscle pump
    d. Do not rely on proper valve closure in the deep veins

16. Increased pressure in the distal venous system seen in secondary varicose veins is due to all of the following except:
    a. Distal obstruction of the venous system
    b. Bidirectional flow in the perforators
    c. Increased pressure in the deep venous system
    d. Increased pressure in the superficial venous system

17. Tissue damage in venous ulcer is:
    a. Fully understood
    b. Due to fibrin accumulation around the capillaries
    c. The trapping of white blood cells in the venules
    d. Still based on theories

18. Vein distension, particularly in the lower extremities during pregnancy, is caused by which of the following?
    a. An increased venous flow velocity
    b. An increased compliance of the veins
    c. Incompetent valves
    d. Compression of the superior vena cava

19. What does a continuous venous flow profile from veins of the lower extremities mean?
    a. The flow is no longer responsive to pressure changes from respiration
    b. It is only seen in pregnancy
    c. It is the result of incompetent valves in the deep system
    d. It is the result of incompetent valves in the superficial system

20. Venous physiology governing blood flow does NOT depend on which of the following?
    a. Venous capacitance
    b. Transmural pressure
    c. Vein compliance
    d. Hydrostatic pressure

FILL-IN-THE-BLANK

1. Veins are known as the capacitance vessels of the body because they act as a _____ for the flow.

2. The cross-sectional area of a distended vein could be _____ larger than the area of the corresponding artery.

3. The fact that veins are usually paired in many area of the body increases the _____ of the vascular system.

4. The most important force affecting the venous system is _____.

5. The hydrostatic pressure is measured by the density of the blood × the acceleration due to gravity × _____.

6. The hydrostatic pressure in an arm raised straight above the head would be _____.

7. Transmural pressure is equal to the _____ between the intravascular pressure in the vein and the pressure in the surrounding tissue.

8. When standing, low-pressure compression stockings have a/an _____ effect in reducing the venous volume.

9. Fluid, which normally moves to the interstitial space of tissue, is usually absorbed by _____ vessels.

10. The pressure exerted by a fluid when there is a difference in the concentrations of solutes across a semipermeable membrane is _____.

11. The _____ plays an important role in the regulation of venous return to the heart by changing the intrathoracic and intra-abdominal pressures.

12. In venous thrombosis of the lower extremities (either partial or complete), the influence of respiration on the intra-abdominal pressure is _____.

13. The calf muscle pump assists in the return of venous flow to the heart when an individual is standing because it works against _____ pressure.

14. Venous reflux in the distal calf during the contraction of the calf muscles under normal conditions is greatly assisted by valve closure in _____.

15. Primary varicose rarely involves the _____ vein.

16. In secondary varicose veins, the flow in the perforators can be _____, which increases the pressure within the superficial system.

17. A serious consequence of venous insufficiency and secondary varicose veins is _____.

18. Increased venous pressure and venous distention _____ cause varicose veins in pregnancy.

19. Typically, varicose veins become _____ with subsequent pregnancies.

20. The venous Doppler signals observed during an ultrasound exam are a direct result of venous _____.

SHORT ANSWER

1. What does increased hydrostatic pressure in the arteries and veins ensure?

2. Why will the pressure in the veins fall below 20 mm Hg during exercise, ensuring an increase of flow across the capillaries?

3. Why is the hydrostatic pressure in an arm raised above the level of the head negative?

4. As the transmural pressure increases, a vein will change to resemble what shapes?

5. What is the condition called when the calf muscle pump works to propel venous flow back to the heart during contraction?

6. What are the main effects of venous hypertension, resulting in difficulty in treatment of venous ulcers?

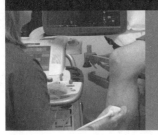

PART 2 • CEREBROVASCULAR

4 The Extracranial Duplex Ultrasound Examination

REVIEW OF GLOSSARY TERMS

MATCHING

Match the key terms with their definitions.

Key Terms

1. ____ Transient ischemic attack
2. ____ Carotid bulb
3. ____ Bruit
4. ____ Spectral analysis
5. ____ Spectral broadening
6. ____ Doppler angle

Definitions

a. Most commonly defined as the angle between the line of the Doppler ultrasound beam and the arterial wall (also referred to as the "angle of insonation"). This is a key variable in the Doppler equation used to calculate flow velocity.

b. An increase in the "width" of the spectral waveform (frequency band) or "filling-in" of the normal clear area under the systolic peak. This represents turbulent blood flow associated with arterial lesions.

c. An episode of stroke-like neurologic symptoms that typically lasts for a few minutes to several hours and then resolves completely. This is caused by temporary interruption of the blood supply to the brain in the distribution of a cerebral artery.

d. A slight dilation involving variable portions of the distal common and proximal internal carotid arteries, often including the origin of the external carotid artery. This is where the baroreceptors assisting in reflex blood pressure control are located. The carotid bulb tends to be most prominent in normal young individuals.

e. Signal processing technique that displays the complete frequency and amplitude content of the Doppler flow signal. The spectral information is usually presented as waveforms with frequency (converted to a velocity scale) on the vertical axis, time on the horizontal axis, and amplitude indicated by a gray scale.

f. An abnormal "blowing" or "swishing" sound heard with a stethoscope while auscultating over an artery such as the carotid. The sound results from vibrations that are transmitted through the tissues when blood flows through a stenotic artery. Whereas the presence of a bruit is a sign of arterial disease, the absence of a bruit is less diagnostic because all stenoses are not associated with bruits.

ANATOMY AND PHYSIOLOGY REVIEW

IMAGE LABELING

Complete the labels in the images that follow.

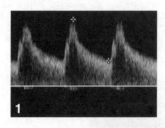 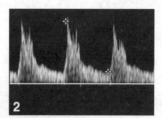

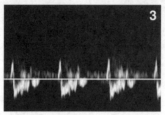

If the following Doppler waveforms were from a normal (nondiseased) internal carotid artery, label what the waveforms would best represent.

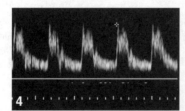 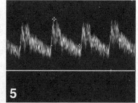

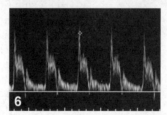

If the following Doppler waveforms were taken from normal (nondiseased) vessels, label the artery that best characterizes the flow based on the waveforms' contours.

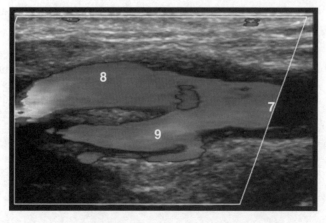

Assuming normal anatomy, label the vessels.

CHAPTER REVIEW

MULTIPLE CHOICE

1. What is the secondary goal of examination of the extracranial carotid artery system by duplex ultrasound?
   a. Identify patients at risk for stroke
   b. Diagnose fibromuscular dysplasia
   c. Document progression of disease
   d. Screen for iatrogenic problems

2. Which of the following transducers can adequately achieve a duplex evaluation of the extracranial cerebrovascular system?
   a. A 7-4 MHz linear array only
   b. A 8-5 MHz curvilinear array only
   c. A 4-1 MHz phased array only
   d. All of the above

3. For a complete duplex evaluation of the extracranial cerebraovascular system, it is strongly recommended that feeding vessels originating from the aortic arch be included and that a bilateral examination be performed. How should the innominate artery be evaluated?
   a. On the right only
   b. On the left only
   c. On both the right and the left
   d. On neither the right nor the left

4. How can the internal and external carotid artery be safely differentiated?
   a. Only by showing that the vessel has no arterial branches
   b. Only by showing that the vessel does not respond to temporal tap with Doppler
   c. Only by demonstrating a low-resistance Doppler spectrum
   d. By showing all of the above

5. What is the most common technique used to identify the vertebral artery?
   a. To view the common carotid artery and angle the transducer slightly posteriorly
   b. To view the subclavian artery and angle the transducer superiorly
   c. To view the basilar artery and angle the transducer inferiorly
   d. To view the vertebral processes and angle the transducer medially

6. In regard to qualifying the appearance of plaque by ultrasound, the use of which of the following terms is discouraged due to poor reliability?
   a. Homogeneous/heterogeneous
   b. Smooth/irregular
   c. Ulcerated
   d. Calcified

7. Which of the following is NOT a nonatherosclerotic lumen reduction that can be seen in the extracranial cerebrovascular system?
   a. Dissection
   b. Arteriovenous fistula
   c. Thrombosis
   d. Stent

8. Which of the following will NOT result in particular symmetrical (i.e., seen in both carotid and sometimes vertebral arterial systems) changes in the Doppler spectra?
   a. Aortic valve or root stenosis
   b. Brain death
   c. Subclavian steal
   d. Intra-aortic balloon pump

9. In a normally hemodynamically low-resistance system or vessel, such as the internal carotid and vertebral arteries, what will a change to high-resistance pattern suggest?
   a. A proximal stenosis or occlusion
   b. A distal stenosis or occlusion
   c. Either A or B
   d. Neither A nor B

10. Reactive hyperemia, as a provocative maneuver used during the duplex evaluation of the extracranial cerebrovascular system, is most important to do what?
    a. Exclude the diagnosis of brain death
    b. Demonstrate a change from latent or partial to complete subclavian steal
    c. Confirm the existence of a unilateral congenital small vertebral artery
    d. Reduce the effect of an intra-aortic balloon pump

11. Which of the following is NOT "sound" advise for sonographers who wish to prevent repetitive stress injuries while scanning?

    a. Be ambidextrous

    b. Arrange bed and equipment to be close to patient

    c. Remain well hydrated during the day

    d. Avoid doing stretching exercises

12. Which of the following does NOT directly influence the Doppler waveform contour?

    a. Flow velocities

    b. Distal resistance

    c. Cardiac output

    d. Vessel compliance

13. Why do Doppler waveforms in the common carotid arteries display a contour suggestive of low-resistance flow?

    a. 70% of its flow supplies the ICA

    b. 90% of it flow supplies the ICA

    c. 70% of it flow supplies the ECA

    d. 90% of it flow supplies the ECA

14. Where does the Doppler waveform contour described as "string sign" usually occur?

    a. Distal to a severe stenosis

    b. Distal to an occlusion

    c. Proximal to a severe stenosis

    d. Proximal to an occlusion

15. Which of the following statements on power Doppler is FALSE?

    a. Represents the amplitude of the Doppler signal instead of frequency shift

    b. Is dependent of the angle of insonation

    c. Does not give information about flow direction

    d. Can detect low-flow states

16. Which of the following did the 2002 panel of experts for consensus on the interpretation of carotid duplex scans NOT recommend?

    a. Lesions of less than 50% diameter reduction should be classified in a single category

    b. Doppler angle should be kept at 60 degree or less but closest to 60

    c. ICA/CCA ratio should be considered a primary diagnostic parameter

    d. Sample volume should be placed at the area of greatest narrowing

17. For an accurate diagnosis of occlusion, what did the 2002 panel of experts for consensus on the interpretation of carotid duplex scans recommend?

    a. The use of gray scale and pulsed Doppler

    b. The use of gray scale or color Doppler

    c. The use of color and power Doppler

    d. The use of gray scale, pulsed Doppler, and color or power Doppler

18. For subclavian steal syndrome or phenomenon to occur, where does a severe stenosis or occlusion need to be present?

    a. The subclavian arteries distal to the vertebral arteries origin

    b. The left subclavian artery or innominate artery proximal to the vertebral arteries origin

    c. The origin of the common carotid arteries

    d. Anywhere in the brachial arteries

19. Which of the following would affect pulsed Doppler spectrum contour in all vessels of the extracranial cerebro arterial system even when no disease is present?

    a. Low-cardiac output

    b. Aortic root stenosis

    c. Intra-aortic balloon pump

    d. All of the above

20. Which of the following statements regarding "flow separation" is FALSE?

    a. It can only occur at the carotid bulb

    b. Results from helical flow pattern

    c. Occurs along the outer wall

    d. Occurs because of reverse flow at low velocities

FILL-IN-THE-BLANK

1. The primary goal of an examination of the extracranial cerebrovascular system by duplex ultrasound is to identify patients at risk for

    _____.

2. Approximately _____ of neck bruits are related to significant stenosis of the internal carotid artery.

3. Lesions or stenoses in the internal carotid arteries _____ present without neurologic symptoms.

4. High-grade stenoses of the internal carotid arteries, as flow restriction lesions, are rarely the primary cause of neurologic symptoms because of _____.

5. RIND, TIA, and CVA are all acronyms describing _____ of neurologic deficits.

6. Flow separation can be seen in the carotid bulb and will be represented by brief flow _____.

7. Transient symptoms manifested as a difficulty to speak are termed as _____.

8. Neurologic deficits lasting between 24 and 72 hours are classified as _____.

9. If significant flow turbulence is noted in the proximal to midright common carotid, it becomes imperative to examine the _____.

10. There are usually two recommended methods to distinguish the internal from the external carotid artery. In the first method, one would recognize the external carotid artery as the artery with _____.

11. In the second method, one would perform _____ to demonstrate the artifact on the Doppler spectrum.

12. The use of a curved or phased array transducer is recommended for the examination of the distal internal carotid arteries, particularly in patients suspected of having _____.

13. The internal characteristics of plaque found in the extracranial cerebrovascular system are usually related to the _____ of the plaque.

14. Dissection of the intima, particularly in common carotid arteries, could be confused with artifacts from the wall of _____.

15. Steal phenomenon occurs because flow (in the cardiovascular system, blood flow) tends to follow the path of _____.

16. "Latent," "hesitant," "alternating," and "complete" are words usually describing the stages of _____.

17. The following terms: "persistence," "priority," "transmit frequency," and "filter" refer to controls available on duplex ultrasound equipment to regulate the appearance of _____.

18. In the presence of significant common carotid stenosis, the ICA/CCA ratio criteria are _____.

19. The NASCET study, although set to evaluate the efficacy of carotid endarterectomy for the prevention of stroke, also prompted the development of _____.

20. Broadening of the Doppler spectrum obtained in a vessel of the extracranial cerebrovascular system is part of interpretation criteria used to classify stenosis developed by _____.

SHORT ANSWER

1. In a normal common carotid artery (free of disease), it is not unusual to detect echoes with apparent motion on B-mode within the vessels lumen. What causes these echoes?

2. The Doppler waveform's contour can be affected systematically in the extracranial cerebrovascular arteries by what artificial cardiac devices?

IMAGE EVALUATION/PATHOLOGY

Review the images and answer the following questions.

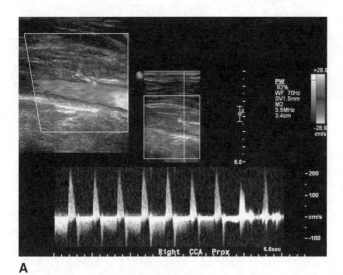

A

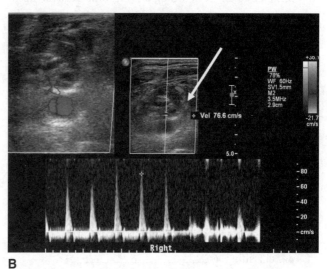

B

1. Based on the characteristics of the Doppler spectrum and the location of the defect, what is the most likely pathology seen in these pictures?

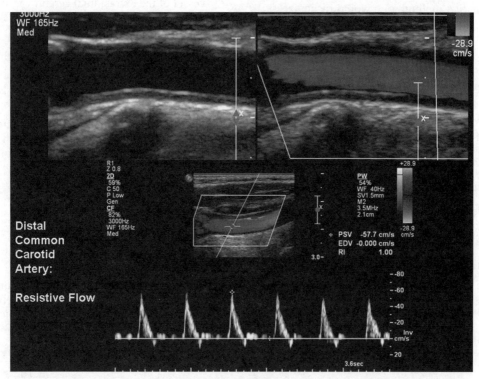

2. Based on the Doppler characteristics seen in this common carotid artery, what is a possible cause?

CASE STUDY

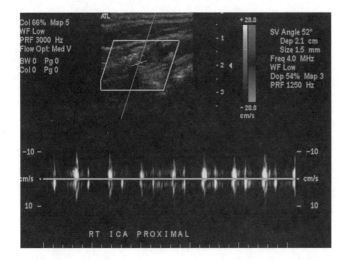

1. Based on the contour of the Doppler waveforms obtained in this proximal right internal carotid artery, what would you expect to find in the remaining of the carotid system for this patient? On the right? On the left (assuming no disease is present)?

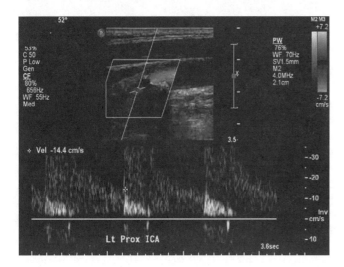

2. Focusing on the Doppler waveforms obtained in this proximal left internal carotid artery and the flow velocities measured (PSV: 14 cm/s, no EDV) and reported, the exam was interpreted as a near occlusion or string sign in the proximal left internal carotid artery. Could there be an alternate interpretation? Why?

The velocities in the common carotid arteries were recorded at: PSV42cm/s EDV 9cm/s on the left and PSV 73 cm/s EDV 27 cm/s on the right. Do these data change your interpretation of the case? Why?

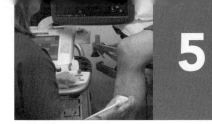

5 Uncommon Pathology of the Carotid System

REVIEW OF GLOSSARY TERMS

MATCHING

Match the key terms with their definitions.

Key Terms

1. _____ Aneurysm
2. _____ Arteritis
3. _____ Carotid body tumor
4. _____ Dissection
5. _____ Fibromuscular dysplasia
6. _____ Intimal flap
7. _____ Pseudoaneurysm
8. _____ Tortuosity

Definitions

a. A dilation of an artery with disruption of one or more layers of the vessel wall causing an expanding hematoma; also called false aneurysm
b. A tear along the inner layer of an artery that results in the splitting or separation of the walls of a blood vessel
c. A localized dilatation of the wall of an artery
d. A benign mass (also called paraganglioma or chemodectoma) of the carotid body, which is a small round mass at the carotid bifurcation
e. A small tear in the wall of a blood vessel resulting in a portion of the intima and part of the media protruding into the lumen of the vessel; this free portion of the blood vessel wall may appear to move with pulsations in flow
f. The quality of being tortuous, winding, twisting
g. Abnormal growth and development of the muscular layer of an artery wall with fibrosis and collagen deposition causing stenosis
h. Inflammation of an artery

CHAPTER REVIEW

MULTIPLE CHOICE

1. A pulsatile mass at the base of the neck may be indicative (and often mistaken) for an aneurysm, when it is most likely tortuosity of which of the following?
   a. The proximal subclavian artery
   b. The proximal vertebral artery
   c. The proximal common carotid
   d. The proximal internal jugular vein

2. Which of the following is NOT a characteristic of the flow in a secondary lumen created by a tear or dissection?
   a. Same direction of flow as in the true lumen
   b. Reverse direction of flow as in the true lumen
   c. An alternate antegrade/retrograde flow pattern in and out of the false lumen
   d. Demonstrate high velocities seen in stenosis

3. What is a likely source of the symptoms in patients under 50 years of age presenting to the vascular lab with symptoms of stroke (without typical risk factors)?
   a. Dissection of one of the carotid vessels
   b. Stenosis due to atherosclerosis
   c. Fibromuscular dysplasia
   d. Tortuous distal ICA with kinking of the vessel

4. What does stenosis occasionally found in false lumen created by dissection often result from?
   a. Atherosclerosis
   b. Thrombosis
   c. Flap
   d. Pseudoaneurysm

5. What is the main feature that should be present for a diagnosis of dissection?
   a. A color pattern clearly showing two flow directions in the lumen
   b. Identifiable thrombus
   c. Atherosclerosis
   d. A hyperechoic (white/bright) line in the lumen of the artery

6. Which condition is repetitive patterns of narrowing and small dilatation in an internal carotid artery, giving the appearance of a "string of beads," typical of?
   a. Dissection
   b. Aneurysms
   c. Fibromuscular dysplasia
   d. Presence of enlarged lymph nodes

7. In a patient with hypertension, incidental diagnosis of fibromuscular dysplasia in the carotid artery system should lead to a follow-up evaluation of which vessel(s)?
   a. The subclavian arteries
   b. The renal arteries
   c. The intracranial vessels
   d. The aorta

8. Which of the following describes a vessel diameter measuring >200% of the diameter of a "normal" section of the ICA or >150% of the CCA?
   a. True aneurysm of carotid vessels
   b. Large carotid bulb
   c. Normal carotid bulb
   d. Pseudoaneurysm

9. Distinguishing a partially thrombosed pseudoaneurysm from a vascularized and enlarged lymph node will be done by observing the flow characteristics of the "feeding" vessel. The pattern of flow in the neck of the pseudoaneurysm will be _____, while the flow in the feeding artery of the lymph node will have _____.
   a. "To and fro," "venous pattern"
   b. "To and fro," "arterial pattern"
   c. "Stenotic," "to and fro"
   d. "Arterial pattern," "stenotic"

10. Why is it important to thoroughly evaluate the vessel wall of the artery where a perforation led to a pseudoaneurysm?
    a. Aliasing is very likely at the area of the perforation
    b. Dissection may occur along the vessel wall
    c. Thrombosis is likely to occur in that area
    d. Plaque is often present in that area

11. When is radiation-induced arterial injury suspected?
    a. The plaque is widespread
    b. The plaque has high echogenicity
    c. The plaque is vascularized
    d. The "plaque" is isolated and located in an atypical area

12. What are the major forms of arteritis found in the carotid system?
    a. Takayasu's disease and temporal arteritis
    b. Giant cell arteritis and FMD
    c. FMD and CBT
    d. None of the above

13. Although giant cells arteritis is typically evaluated by ultrasound in the superficial temporal artery, which of the following can this pathology affect?
    a. The facial artery
    b. The occipital artery
    c. The internal maxillary artery
    d. All of the above

14. Why is it crucial to survey the entire visible length of the vessel when evaluating the superficial temporal artery for signs of temporal arteritis?
    a. The inflamed area is not continuous
    b. The vessel is often tortuous
    c. Dissections are often present locally
    d. Areas of dilatation are present locally

15. A 30-year-old female presents to the vascular lab with decreased radial pulses and upper extremities claudication. What would you suspect?
    a. Takayasu's disease
    b. Giant cell arteritis
    c. Carotid body tumor
    d. Spontaneous dissection

16. A 60-year-old female presents to the vascular lab with history of headaches and tenderness in the temporal area as well as jaw claudication. What would you suspect?
    a. Takayasu's disease
    b. Carotid body tumor
    c. Giant cell arteritis
    d. Spontaneous dissection

17. A 25-year-old male involved in competitive bicycle racing presents in the vascular lab with symptoms of headaches and subtle neurological changes. What would you suspect?
    a. Giant cell arteritis
    b. Spontaneous dissection
    c. Takayasu's disease
    d. Carotid body tumor

18. A 75-year-old male with long-lasting history of COPD presents in the vascular lab for evaluation of his carotid arteries. An incidental mass is visualized at the carotid bifurcation on the right side. What would you suspect?
    a. Spontaneous dissection
    b. Carotid body tumor
    c. Giant cell arteritis
    d. Takayasu's disease

19. You are asked to evaluate a pulsatile neck mass in an 80-year-old female with recent placement of a central line in the right internal jugular vein. What would you suspect?
    a. A pseudoaneurysm
    b. An enlarged lymph node
    c. A carotid body tumor
    d. A dissection

20. A 50-year-male with history of non-Hodgkin lymphoma treated with radiation presents in the vascular lab with some neurological changes. What would you suspect?
    a. Carotid body tumor
    b. Enlarged lymph nodes
    c. Radiation-induced arterial disease
    d. Dissection

FILL-IN-THE-BLANK

1. Application of flow velocities criteria for the accurate evaluation of a tortuous internal carotid artery is difficult. It is therefore recommended that particular attention be placed on the image with and without _____ to identify pathologies.

2. A dissection of an arterial wall may create what is commonly referred to as a _____ lumen.

3. One of the main challenges in evaluating a tortuous internal carotid artery is that the "twists" and "turns" may overlap _____.

4. It is important to obtain a thorough medical or lifestyle history to evaluate for subtle trauma to the neck in patients presenting with _____.

5. A "to-and-fro" pattern of flow seen in a false lumen created by a dissection should suggest an _____.

6. Fibromuscular dysplasia affects predominantly _____.

7. One of the best "tools" available on duplex ultrasound to clearly depict the "string of beads" appearance associated with fibromuscular dysplasia in the internal carotid artery is

   _____.

8. The Doppler spectrum in the arteries found within a carotid body tumor will typically display _____ resistance characteristic.

9. Penetrating trauma to the neck, presence of a bypass graft in the carotid system, or history of endarterectomy may (although rare) lead to the formation of _____.

10. The area of highest narrowing seen with radiation-induced arterial injury tends to be at the _____ end of the stenotic area.

11. A long, homogeneous narrowing typically seen in the subclavian artery of a young female patient would suggest _____.

12. In a transverse view, a "halo" surrounding the outer layer of the facial artery may suggest

    _____.

13. Two clearly different Doppler spectrum seen as Doppler sampling on each side of a "white" line in an arterial lumen suggests _____.

14. A focal plaque without the typical appearance of atherosclerosis and located in the midright common carotid artery may suggest _____.

15. Inflammation of an artery, which may result in the breakdown of the structure of the arterial wall, is generally termed as _____.

16. Injury to the vasa vasorum, located in the media of arterial wall and resulting in fibrosis of the portion of the wall, is the basis for lesions seen with

    _____.

17. Typically, nonmalignant paragangliomas of the neck are also called _____.

18. An abnormal growth of smooth muscle cells in the media of the internal carotid artery has been shown to be the underlying pathologic mechanism of

    _____.

19. It is believed that possibly one-fourth of the adult population present with some degree of the following finding bilaterally _____, predominantly in the distal internal carotid arteries.

20. To ensure that velocity changes (particularly sudden increases) in a tortuous vessel are the result of a stenosis rather than sudden changes in direction of flow, one should thoroughly examined the vessels in

    _____.

SHORT ANSWER

1. What is prominent tortuosity at the origin of the right or left carotid artery or at the level of the innominate artery often mistaken for and why?

2. To distinguish between aliasing due to a stenosis from aliasing due to tortuosity of a vessel, special attention should be paid to what?

IMAGE EVALUATION/PATHOLOGY

Review the images and answer the following questions.

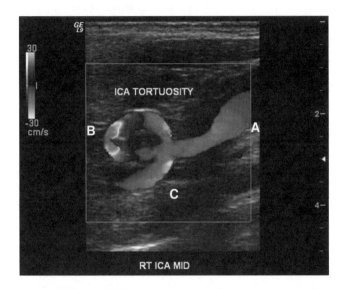

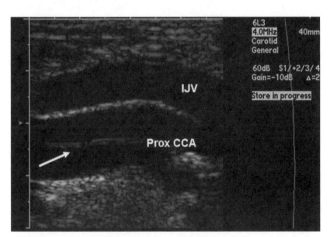

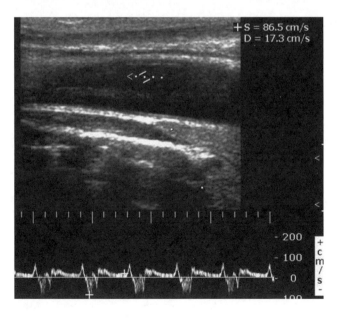

1. Describe the flow direction in area A, B, and C (in relation to the transducer)

2. In area B, how would you label the mosaic of color seen?

3. What Doppler angle would probably need to be used in each area—A, B, and C—to record velocities (estimate)?

4. What is the arrow most likely pointing to?

5. The Doppler spectrum seen here (in the context of the pathology depicted) would suggest that the sample volume is positioned in?

CASE STUDY

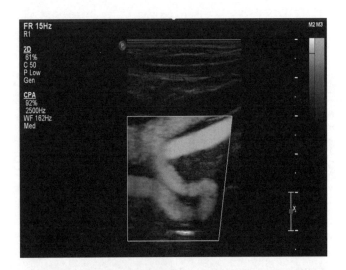

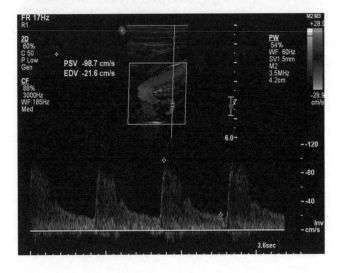

1. These two images were taken at the same level in a patient. Which artery is most likely depicted in these images? Why? Which techniques are used in each image to show flow? What is the advantage of using each technique? The flow velocities were recorded as: PSV: 98.7 cm/s, EDV: 21.6 cm/s. What is missing? Discuss the accuracy of the data.

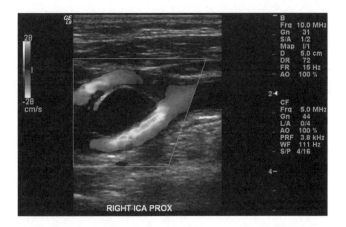

RIGHT ICA PROX

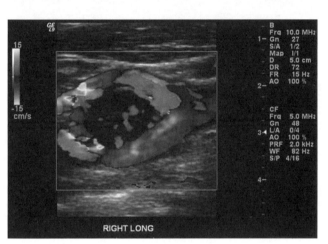

RIGHT LONG

2. These images were taken at the level of the bifurcation of internal and external carotid arteries. What rather uncommon pathology is most likely represented in this image? Describe the relevant points leading to your conclusion. Between image 1 and image 2, the sonographer changed one of the settings for color display. Explain the rationale for the choice. What alternate tool could have been used? What would you expect to find in the history (medical, lifestyle) for this patient to explain the pathology seen here? In other words, what are risk factors or underlying conditions commonly associated with this pathology?

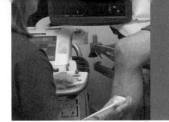

6 Ultrasound Following Surgery and Intervention

REVIEW OF GLOSSARY TERMS

MATCHING

Match the key terms with their definitions.

Key Terms

1. _____ Carotid artery stenting

2. _____ Carotid endarterectomy

3. _____ Arteriotomy

4. _____ Instent restenosis

5. _____ Polytetrafluoroethyene

Definitions

a. A surgical procedure during which the carotid artery is opened and plaque is removed in order to restore normal luminal diameter

b. A narrowing of the lumen of a stent, which causes a stenosis

c. A surgical incision through the wall of an artery into the lumen

d. Abbreviated PTFE, a synthetic graft material used to create grafts and blood vessel patches; a common brand name is Gore-tex

e. A catheter-based procedure in which a metal mesh tube is deployed into an artery to keep it open, following balloon angioplasty to dilate a stenosis

CHAPTER REVIEW

MULTIPLE CHOICE

1. A typical carotid endarterectomy procedure involves a longitudinal arteriotomy from where to where?

   a. A normal distal ECA to the bulb and ICA

   b. A normal proximal CCA to ICA

   c. A normal proximal ICA to the bulb

   d. A normal distal portion of ICA toward the CCA

2. Which of the following is NOT a common problem leading to stenosis at the level of the arteriotomy performed during endarterectomy?

   a. Female gender

   b. Narrowing due to sutures

   c. Retained plaque

   d. Hyperplastic response

3. Why does the eversion technique used more often for carotid endarterectomy result in fewer complications for stenosis due to suture?

   a. The technique does not require a patch

   b. The sutures are not on the superficial wall of the artery

   c. The ICA is reverted to its original position after the procedure

   d. The sutures are at the widened area of the bulb

4. When evaluating an endarterectomy site within 48 hours of the surgical procedure, one should be mindful of preventing infection by using all of the following EXCEPT:

   a. Using sterile gel

   b. Leaving the sterile dressing in place

   c. Using sterile pads

   d. Using sterile transducer cover

5. Because of limitations in evaluating the vessels following an endarterectomy, what should the sonographer pay particular attention to?

   a. Quality of flow in the vertebral arteries

   b. Quality of flow in the proximal ICA

   c. Quality of flow in the distal ICA

   d. Quality of flow in the contralateral ICA

6. Which of the following may NOT be associated with vein patch rupture?

   a. Pseudoaneurysm

   b. Hematoma

   c. Infection

   d. Extravasation

7. What is a perivascular fluid collection above an irregular buckling of a patch an indication of?

   a. Active infection

   b. Pseudoaneurysm

   c. Hematoma

   d. Patch rupture

8. What is stenosis at the CEA site is usually considered to result from more than 24 months after an endarterectomy?

   a. Neointimal hyperplasia

   b. Thrombosis

   c. Atherosclerotic process

   d. Intimal flap

9. What did a significant result of the CREST and ICSS studies show?

   a. CEA results in more stroke than CAS

   b. CEA results in more restenosis than CAS

   c. CAS results in more stroke than CEA

   d. CAS results in more restenosis than CEA

10. Where was the ICSS study conducted mainly?

    a. Canada

    b. The United States

    c. Asia

    d. Europe

11. Which artery is most often used for catheter insertion for CAS?

    a. The popliteal artery

    b. The common femoral artery

    c. The brachial artery

    d. The common carotid artery

12. What is the guidewire used for CAS usually first used to deploy and position?

    a. The embolic protection device

    b. The balloon catheter

    c. The stent catheter

    d. The sheath

13. Stent distortion has been reported with mechanical forces on the neck from all of the following EXCEPT:

    a. Head tilting

    b. Coughing

    c. Neck rotations

    d. Swallowing

14. For maximal efficacy, how far should a stent length extend proximal and distal to the lesion?
    a. 2 mm
    b. 0.5 mm
    c. 5 mm
    d. 10 mm

15. What would be the result of coverage of the origin of the ECA during and after stent deployment?
    a. Not be a contraindication
    b. Be of great consideration
    c. Lead to compromise of flow
    d. Cause dissection

16. Why does neointimal hyperplasia seen in CAS differ from the phenomenon seen in CEA?
    a. Stents only lead to a single intimal injury
    b. Stents are implanted foreign object
    c. Restenosis is variable with stents
    d. Increased risk of dissection

17. What should diffuse proliferative narrowing within a stent without increased flow velocities do?
    a. Not be a source of concern
    b. Lead the sonographer to explore technical errors
    c. Be suggestive of type V restenosis
    d. Lead to increased follow-up

18. What has the most important predictor (as a risk factor) for type IV restenosis been shown to be?
    a. Atherosclerosis
    b. Smoking
    c. Diabetes
    d. Hypertension

19. What does type I instant restenosis of stents involve?
    a. The stent border
    b. The entire stent
    c. The ICA proximal to the stent
    d. The ICA distal to the stent

20. Which of the following is true of postprocedural elevation of velocities in CAS?
    a. It is always a sign of restenosis
    b. It is not as frequent as in CEA
    c. It is not a sign of restenosis
    d. It is the result of great compliance of the stent

FILL-IN-THE-BLANK

1. Clear and standardized criteria have yet to be established for the evaluation of carotid artery stenting by duplex ultrasound because CAS is still in a period of _____.

2. The solution most often used to reduce the potential for procedure-induced stenosis with carotid endarterectomy involves the suturing of a _____.

3. Most problems arising after a carotid endarterectomy will be located at the _____ border of the arteriotomy.

4. A vein used as surgical patch for carotid endarterectomy will often be everted such as to provide a double layer of vessel wall, with the _____ of the vein facing the lumen of the artery.

5. Eversion technique for endarterectomy involves a complete _____ of the ICA and ECA at the level of the carotid bulb.

6. It is not unusual to find entrapped air directly above the CEA site. In such case, the sonographer could image the vessels using a more _____ approach.

7. Synthetic patches are usually more _____ than autogenous patches.

8. Stenosis seen after 1 month and within 24 months postendarterectomy is usually the result of _____.

9. The role of the sonographer in the postprocedural evaluation for carotid stenting involves considering a path for safe _____ insertion.

10. Until the results of the CREST and ICSS studies, CAS was mostly recommended for _____ patients with high perioperative risks.

11. Postprocedural complications of CAS are not limited to the carotid vessels but can also be seen in the _____ artery.

12. The more common use of stents has resulted in different complications than with CEA. Although fractures per se are rare, the stents are under many _____ forces.

13. Fracture of stents has been demonstrated with higher incidence when the underlying plaque was _____.

14. The natural history of deployed stents and the occurrence of late complications are _____ documented.

15. The single greatest concern of poststent evaluation is _____.

16. The most common type of instant restenosis found with CAS is _____.

17. When using flow velocity criteria, the primary discriminator of significant restenosis in CAS is _____.

18. A high-grade restenosis seen in CAS should correlate with PSV of _____.

19. Dense circumferential calcification is of particular concerns with CAS because it _____ balloon expansion.

20. Reintervention for either CEA or CAS would be warranted if the treated lesion leads to _____.

SHORT ANSWER

1. What differences exist in the evaluation of carotid endarterectomy and carotid artery stenting by duplex ultrasound?

2. What are surgical patches for carotid endarterectomy typically made from?

3. Once the stent has been placed and allowed to self expand, what happens next?

4. What should sonographers use to evaluate stents for evidence of diffuse narrowing?

5. When would re-exploration of CEA or CAS be necessary?

IMAGE EVALUATION/PATHOLOGY

Review the images and answer the following questions.

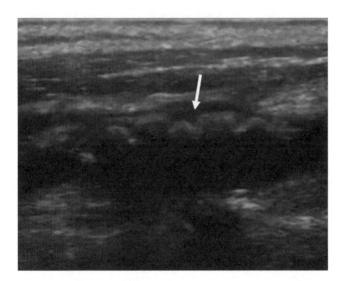

1. What is the pathology suggested in this image of a Dacron patch in a carotid artery?

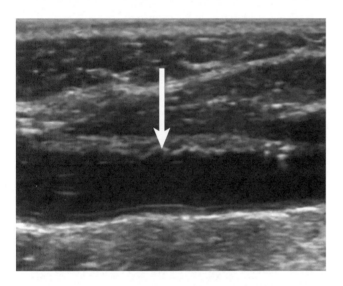

2. In this image taken on a follow-up exam postcarotid endarterectomy, what is the most likely structure outlined by the arrow?

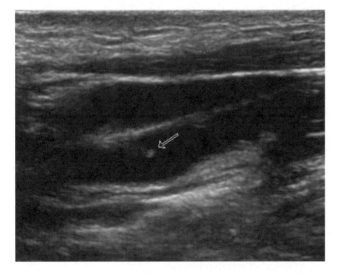

3. What does the white arrow in this image most likely represent?

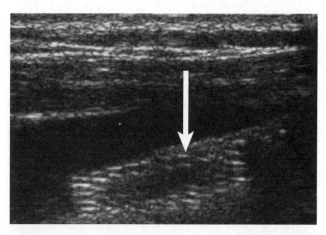

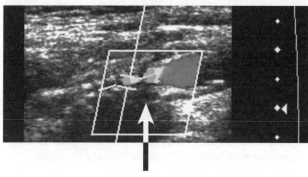

4. What does the arrow (below the level of the Doppler sampling) in this stent represent?

5. What does the arrow point to?

CASE STUDY

1. A 55-year-old male with long-standing history of type I diabetes mellitus was recently treated for a hemodynamically significant stenosis of his right internal carotid artery, with a stent. The procedure was done on May 2. The patient is scheduled for a follow-up ultrasound of the stented carotid a month after the procedure.

2. A 78-year-old female has undergone a left carotid endarterectomy 1 month prior to presenting in your vascular lab. The procedure was done at another facility, and the notes are not available. The patient has been referred by a physician based on concerns from her son that his mother seems to still experience some pain and swelling on the left side of her neck.

On June 5th, the patient reports to the vascular lab for a follow-up exam. The sonographer notes flow velocities in the 150 cm/s range within the stent (versus velocities of 90 cm/s in the ICA proximal and distal to the stent). What should be considered in regard to these flow velocities? What should be excluded in this first postprocedure exam?

Because the patient is a female, what should you consider about the procedure done?

What could be the complications to consider with the use of a patch on an endarterectomy site?

On December 12, the patient reports to the vascular lab for a 6 month follow-up. His physician noted a bruit during physical examination the previous day. What should be considered (based on the patient's medical history)? What should be recommended for follow-up based on results on this exam?

When evaluating swelling from fluid accumulation from inflammation or infection, how can you distinguish swelling from the incision site from infection at the patch level?

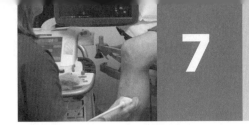

7 Intracranial Cerebrovascular Examination

REVIEW OF GLOSSARY TERMS

MATCHING

Match the key terms with their definitions.

Key Terms

1. _____ Transcranial Doppler

2. _____ Transcranial duplex imaging

3. _____ Circle of Willis

4. _____ Vasospasm

5. _____ Collateral

6. _____ Pulsatility

7. _____ Lindegaard ratio

8. _____ Sviri ratio

Definitions

a. A noninvasive test on the intracranial cerebral blood vessels that uses ultrasound and provides both an image of the blood vessels and a graphical display of the velocities within the vessels

b. Expressed as Gosling's pulsatility index (peak systolic velocity minus end-diastolic velocity divided by the time-averaged peak velocity)

c. A vessel that parallels another vessel; a vessel that is important to maintain blood flow around another stenotic or occluded vessel

d. Middle cerebral artery (MCA) mean velocity divided by the submandibular internal carotid artery (ICA) mean velocity. This ratio is useful in differentiating increased volume flow from decreased diameter when high velocities are encountered in the MCA or intracranial ICA.

e. Ratio calculation used to determine vasospasm from hyperdynamic flow in the posterior circulation. The bilateral vertebral artery velocities taken at the atlas loop are added together and averaged. This averaged velocity is then divided into the highest basilar mean velocity.

f. A roughly circular anastomosis of arteries located at the base of the brain

g. A sudden constriction in a blood vessel, causing a restriction in blood flow

h. A noninvasive test that uses ultrasound to measure the velocity of blood flow through the intracranial cerebral vessels

ANATOMY AND PHYSIOLOGY REVIEW

IMAGE LABELING

Complete the labels in the images that follow.

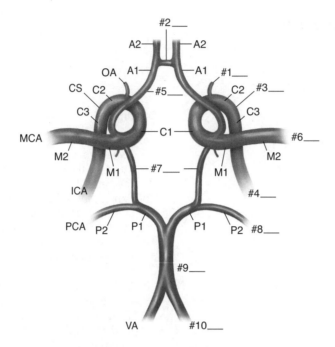

Circle of Willis and branches.

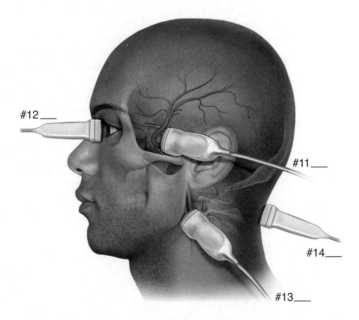

Four approaches used for intracranial exams.

CHAPTER REVIEW

MULTIPLE CHOICE

1. What is the range of the average diameter of basal cerebral arteries?
   a. 1 to 3 cm
   b. 1 to 3 mm
   c. 2 to 4 cm
   d. 2 to 4 mm

2. It is estimated that 18% to 54% of individuals display variations at the level of the circle of Willis. Which of the following is NOT one of these variations?
   a. Variation of number of arteries
   b. Variation of caliber of vessels
   c. Variation of the course of vessels
   d. Variation of the origin of branches

3. What are the parasellar, genu, and supraclinoid segments part of?
   a. The carotid siphon
   b. The posterior cerebral artery
   c. The middle cerebral artery
   d. The anterior cerebral artery

4. Which of the following statement about the anterior cerebral arteries is FALSE?
   a. The anterior communicating artery is located above the optic chiasm
   b. Both arteries (right and left) are frequently identical
   c. Both arteries communicate via the anterior communicating artery
   d. Both arteries first course medially to the internal carotid arteries

5. Which of the following is a typical characteristic of a nonimaging transducer for transcranial Doppler?
   a. 1 to 2 MHz pulsed wave
   b. 1 to 2 MHz continuous wave
   c. >4 MHz pulsed wave
   d. >4 MHz continuous wave

6. What is the Doppler frequency range in standard duplex imaging system for transcranial?
   a. 1 to 2 MHz
   b. 2 to 3 MHz
   c. 4 MHz
   d. >4MHz

7. What is the initial target vessel to be explored through the transtemporal acoustic window?
   a. The ACA
   b. The PCA
   c. The MCA
   d. The carotid siphon

8. What are the Lindegaard and the BA/VA ratios both useful for the categorization of?
   a. Distal ICA stenosis
   b. Subarachnoid hemorrhaging
   c. Dissections
   d. Vasospasm

9. What does the relation, MCA>ACA>PCA=BA=VA, represents?
   a. Relative flow velocities
   b. Relative size of the vessels
   c. Relative direction of flow in the vessels
   d. Relation to the acoustic window

10. Which of the following is NOT a criterion used for the identification of vessels or vessel segments in the intracranial circulation?
    a. The direction of flow in relation to the transducer
    b. The diameter of the vessel
    c. The sample volume depth
    d. The vessel flow velocity

11. Which of the following is a quality of the accurate calculation of flow velocities with TCD?
    a. Independent of the pitch of the signal
    b. Based on a measured angle
    c. Based on patient's cooperation
    d. Operator dependent

12. Which of the following is NOT a primary diagnostic feature of the Doppler signals for evaluation of intracranial vessels?
    a. Changes in various ratios from established criteria
    b. Changes in velocity from established criteria
    c. Changes in flow pulsatility from established standards
    d. Changes in flow direction from established standards

13. Which of the following collateral pathways will NOT show direct evidence of significant carotid artery disease?
    a. Crossover collateral through ACoA
    b. Posterior to anterior flow through PCoA
    c. Leptomeningeal collateralization
    d. Reversed ophthalmic artery

14. Which of the statement below is NOT part of the five primary criteria used to identify intracranial arterial segment?
    a. Flow direction
    b. Pulsatility index
    c. Sample volume depth
    d. Window/approach used

15. A limited transcranial Doppler or transcranial duplex imaging exam could be ordered for all of the following EXCEPT:
    a. Evaluate for sickle cell anemia
    b. Monitor microembolism during endarterectomy
    c. Follow-up for vasospasm
    d. Evaluate single vessel patency

16. Which of the following statements regarding the use (and advantages) of audio signals during TCD and TCDI is FALSE?
    a. Nuances in signal can be heard before they can be seen on the Doppler spectrum
    b. High-velocity signals could be missed by turbulent flow on the Doppler spectrum
    c. Audio signals can help in redirecting the sonographer in the acquisition of Doppler spectrum
    d. TCDI does not have audio capability

17. Which of the following is the Atlas loop approach used for?
    a. Visualizing the internal carotid siphon
    b. Visualizing the distal vertebral arteries
    c. Obtaining data to characterize basilar artery vasospasm
    d. Alternative window to the foramen magnum approach

18. To ensure patient safety when using the transorbital approach, which technical setting should you always address?
    a. Decrease the acoustic intensity
    b. Decrease the velocity scale
    c. Increase the Doppler gain
    d. Increase the color Doppler scale

19. At a depth of approximately 65 mm from the transtemporal window, with a Doppler sample gate of 5 to 10 mm, you should obtain two Doppler spectra (one on each side of the baseline). What do these Doppler spectra correspond to?
    a. Siphon/MCA
    b. Right MCA/left MCA
    c. ACA/ACoA
    d. MCA/ACA

20. When is evidence of vasospasm usually seen following subarachnoid hemorrhaging?
    a. 3 to 4 days after the bleed started
    b. 6 to 8 days after the bleed started
    c. 2 to 4 weeks after the bleed started
    d. 6 to 8 weeks after the bleed started

FILL-IN-THE-BLANK

1. On average, the center of the Circle of Willis is approximately the size of a _____.

2. The anterior intracranial arterial circulation is formed as a continuation of the _____.

3. In 18% to 27% of the population, the posterior cerebral arteries receive blood flow (at least partly) from the _____.

4. The anterior inferior cerebellar and superior cerebellar arteries are branches of the _____.

5. The posterior inferior cerebellar arteries are typically branches of the _____.

6. The best acoustic window to insonate the vertebral and basilar arteries is through the _____.

7. On nonimaging transcranial Doppler, a visual colored roadmap of vessels is possible because of the addition of _____.

8. Independently of the technique use (TCD or TCDI), the documentation of data obtained on intracranial arteries is based on _____.

9. All of the arteries examined during a TCD or TCDI examination supply the brain except the _____.

10. When the transducer is placed 1.25 in below the mastoid process and posterior to the sternocleidomastoid muscle, the technique is called the _____ approach.

11. The Gosling index expresses the _____ of the Doppler signal.

12. The MCA mean velocity divided by the submandibular ICA mean velocity represents the calculation for the _____ ratio.

13. Ipsilateral increased velocities observed in the ACA and PCA with a significant stenosis or occlusion of the MCA is a result of _____ collateralization.

14. Evaluation of the MCA from a temporal window with a more posterior location will require aiming the transducer _____.

15. The location at the temporal window resulting in a neutral orientation of the transducer to evaluate the MCA is _____.

16. A "fifth" acoustic window is sometimes used for transcranial examination; this window is the _____.

17. The two anterior cerebral arteries are usually connected by an anterior communicating artery at this level _____.

18. The frequency found in most TCD (nonimaging) transducers is typically _____.

19. The imaging frequency found in most TCDI (duplex) transducers is typically _____.

20. The Doppler frequency found in most TCDI (duplex) transducers is typically _____.

SHORT ANSWER

1. With transcranial Doppler, why is spectral broadening unavoidable?

2. Why are velocities acquired during a transcranial exam usually referred to as mean velocities?

3. What are the main quantitative values used for diagnostic purposes in a transcranial exam?

4. All Doppler spectra obtained from examination of intracranial arteries should have low-resistance characteristics except those obtained in what?

5. Because of individual variations of the temporal window, the area is often subdivided into what?

IMAGE EVALUATION/PATHOLOGY

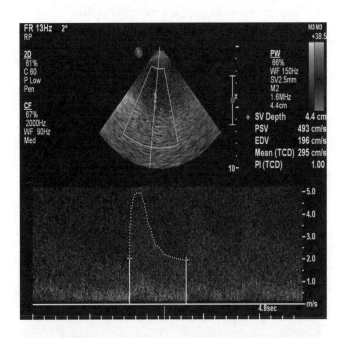

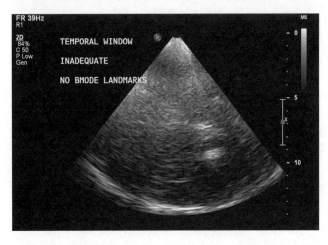

1. What do the Doppler spectrum profile and the flow velocities obtained in the right MCA suggest?

2. In this image, why would the examination be limited and diagnosis difficult? Which arteries of the circle of Willis would you not be able to obtain information for?

CASE STUDY

1. You are asked to evaluate a 25-year-old male, post–motor vehicle accident with head injury, currently in critical condition in the intensive care unit. Your lab does not usually handle neurological exams, so you do not have a set protocol for these exams. What would be the main consideration in this case? To set up an efficient protocol that will allow for sequential exams, the main arteries to monitor would be at a minimum. Which approach would you use? How would you set up your schedule to monitor this patient?

2. A 75-year-old female is seen for follow-up in the vascular lab. Previous exams have documented severe stenosis of the distal right common carotid artery. The patient has remained mostly asymptomatic. In this exam, the result shows a complete occlusion of the right common carotid artery. She still does not recall much changes or symptoms. Flow is noted in the ICA and ECA. Her physician orders a transcranial study to assess the intracranial circulation. What would you expect the flow (particularly in regard to direction of flow) to be in the ICA and ECA? What typical collateral pathway could have lead to this redistribution of flow? What would you expect the flow direction to be in the main vessel from that collateral pathway?

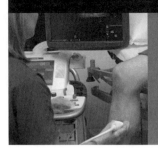

8 Indirect Assessment of Arterial Disease

REVIEW OF GLOSSARY TERMS

MATCHING

Match the key terms with their definitions.

Key Terms

1. _____ Claudication

2. _____ Rest pain

3. _____ Ankle–brachial index

4. _____ Plethysmography

5. _____ Photoplethysmography

6. _____ Raynaud's disease

7. _____ Thoracic outlet syndrome

8. _____ Allen test

Definitions

a. Pain in the extremity without exercise or activity, thus, "at rest," can occur in the toes, foot, or ankle area

b. Pain in muscle groups brought on by exercise or activity that recedes with cessation of activity; can occur in the calf, thigh, and buttock

c. The ratio of ankle systolic pressure to brachial systolic pressure

d. Vasospasm of the digital arteries brought on by exposure to cold; can be caused by numerous etiologies

e. An indirect physiologic test that detects changes in back-scattered infrared light as an indicator of tissue perfusion

f. An indirect physiologic test that measures the change in volume or impedance in a whole body, organ, or limb

g. Compression of the brachial nerve plexus, subclavian artery, or subclavian vein at the region where these structures exit the thoracic cavity and course peripherally toward the arm

h. A series of maneuvers testing the digital perfusion of the hand while compressing and releasing the radial and ulnar arteries

ANATOMY AND PHYSIOLOGY REVIEW

IMAGE LABELING

Complete the labels in the images that follow.

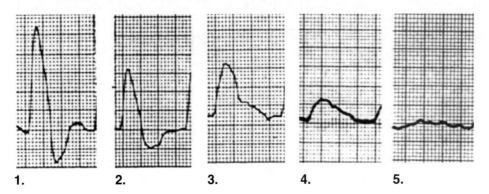

1.   2.   3.   4.   5.

Various Doppler waveforms

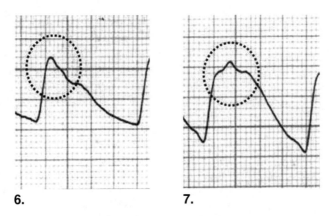

6.   7.

Digital PPG waveforms.

CHAPTER REVIEW

MULTIPLE CHOICE

1. The most common method to calculate ABI is to relate which of the following?
   a. The lowest pressure at the ankle to the lowest systolic pressure of the right or left brachial artery
   b. The highest pressure at the ankle to the highest systolic pressure of the right or left brachial artery
   c. The highest or the lowest pressure at the ankle to the highest systolic pressure of the right or left brachial artery
   d. The highest pressure at the ankle to the lowest systolic pressure of the right or left brachial artery

2. Which of the following statements about intermittent claudication is FALSE?
   a. Pain with exercise is relieved by rest
   b. It can be asymptomatic at rest
   c. ABI values are generally between 0.5 and 1.3
   d. ABI value can never be greater than 1.3

3. Which of the following statements regarding the importance of early assessment of the presence of PAD is FALSE?
   a. Patients are at increased risk for cardiovascular mortality
   b. Patients are at increased risk for cardiovascular morbidity
   c. Patients will eventually require an amputation
   d. PAD is a marker for systemic arterial damage

4. Progression of PAOD can be established on follow-up of patients by physical exam and clinical history because the patient may describe all of the following EXCEPT:
   a. Diminution of walking distance
   b. Increase of recovery time
   c. Skin and nails changes
   d. Resolution of pain by changing position

5. Severe PAOD can be suspected with all of the following EXCEPT:
   a. Leg pain while sitting
   b. Skin discoloration and scaling
   c. Claudication pain after less than 50-ft walk
   d. Constant forefoot pain

6. Thoracic outlet syndromes can include all of the following presentations EXCEPT:
   a. Pain with arm in neutral position
   b. Neurological pain
   c. Edema of the arm and forearm
   d. Pain with arm elevated above head

7. The techniques commonly used for indirect testing of arterial perfusion in the thigh and leg include all of the following EXCEPT:
   a. Plethysmography
   b. Photoplethysmography
   c. Doppler waveforms analysis
   d. Segmental systolic pressure

8. To ensure accuracy of data, particularly for recording of segmental systolic pressures, how long should the patient be allowed to rest?
   a. 5 to 10 minutes
   b. 10 to 15 minutes
   c. 20 minutes
   d. Does not need to rest

9. Which of the following should the cuff size be to ensure accuracy of data obtained with systolic pressure determination?
   a. A 12-cm wide cuff at the upper arm
   b. A 10-cm wide cuff at the ankle
   c. Between 10% and 15% wider than the diameter of the limb segment
   d. Twenty percent wider than the diameter of the limb segment

10. Systolic pressures can be falsely determined in the lower extremities with all of the following EXCEPT:
    a. The cuff is too narrow
    b. The deflation rate is too fast
    c. The limb segment is elevated above the heart
    d. The dorsalis pedis artery is used to listen to the signal

11. What will the use of a 4-cuffs versus a 3-cuffs method to estimate arterial disease in the lower extremities help determine?
    a. If disease is present at the distal femoral level
    b. If disease is present at the proximal femoral level
    c. If disease is present at the iliofemoral level
    d. If disease is present at the popliteal level

12. Which of the following is a clear diagnostic criteria to estimate disease between two limb segments when using systolic pressure determination?
    a. A drop of more than 30 mm Hg between the proximal and immediate distal segment
    b. An increase of more than 30 mm Hg between the proximal and immediate distal segment
    c. A drop of 50 mm Hg between the proximal and immediate distal segment
    d. An increase of 50 mm Hg between the proximal and immediate distal segment

13. Which of the following is NOT a common method to induce symptoms with exercise in a patient suspected to have arterial insufficiency but relatively normal results at rest?

    a. Using a treadmill for walking with a set protocol

    b. Having the patient walk at own pace until symptoms occur

    c. Having the patient perform heel raises until symptoms occur

    d. Raising the limb above the heart while the patient is supine on the exam table

14. Which of the following is NOT one of the main advantages of pulse volume recording (PVR)?

    a. Records overall segment perfusion

    b. Can give data even with calcified arteries

    c. Is easy and quick to perform

    d. Is not concerned with flow direction

15. The most convenient (and reliable) technique to obtain digital pressures is using a small cuff with:

    a. PVR

    b. PPG

    c. CW Doppler

    d. PW Doppler

16. What is the most convenient technique to record changes of arterial insufficiency with thoracic outlet syndrome with a specific (and sometimes tailored) set of maneuvers?

    a. PVR on a limb segment

    b. CW Doppler at the brachial artery

    c. Pressure recordings at the brachial artery

    d. PPG on a digit

17. What is the typical skin color changes (in the hands and fingers) from room temperature to exposure to cold temperature and ending with rewarming?

    a. White, blue, red

    b. Red, blue, white

    c. Blue, white, red

    d. Blue, red, white

18. The Allen test should be performed before all of the following procedures could be done EXCEPT:

    a. Creation of an arteriovenous fistula

    b. Creation of a dialysis access

    c. Harvest of the cephalic vein for bypass

    d. Harvest of the radial artery for a coronary bypass

19. The Allen test is typically performed by placing a PPG sensor on the middle or index finger to record digit perfusion while:

    a. The radial and ulnar arteries are compressed concomitantly

    b. The radial and ulnar arteries are compressed sequentially

    c. The radial artery is compressed individually

    d. The ulnar artery is compressed individually

20. Using PPG sensor on a digit demonstrating signs of increased vasospasm from primary Raynaud's disease, what characteristic will the waveform typically display?

    a. An anacrotic notch in systole

    b. An anacrotic notch in late diastole

    c. A dicrotic notch in systole

    d. A dicrotic notch in diastole

FILL-IN-THE-BLANK

1. Most often, symptoms of arterial disease are described as "intermittent" claudication because the symptoms occur _____.

2. Symptoms observed or described with intermittent claudication can determine the site of disease because the disease is _____ to the site of symptoms.

3. Muscular pain localized in the calf brought on by walking would most likely be due to disease located at the level of the _____.

4. Elevation pallor and dependent rubor is usually observed with _____ arterial disease.

5. The cause of primary Raynaud's disease is

    _____.

6. PAOD in the upper extremities is

    _____.

7. The ideal positioning of patients for indirect arterial testing should take great care that all extremities are not elevated above _____.

8. For recording of accurate segmental systolic pressures, it is important not only to allow the patient to rest before the test, but also to ensure that _____ is appropriately sized for the limb segment.

9. An ideal cuff deflation rate for accurately determining the return of Doppler signal when measuring systolic pressure at any segment should be approximately _____.

10. The lowest limit of an ABI to be considered within normal range at rest is _____.

11. When ABIs appear abnormally high and disease is suspected (by signs, symptoms, or the results from other tests), a primary cautionary measure would be to reassess the brachial pressure because it may have _____.

12. When using a 4-cuffs method, the two thigh cuffs will require a _____ inflation pressure to exert compression of the underlying arteries.

13. Under normal condition (absence of disease), the high-thigh pressure using a 4-cuffs method will usually be at least _____ greater than the normal brachial pressure.

14. In the upper extremities, using segmental pressure as a diagnostic criteria, significant disease will be likely when a drop of at least _____ is recorded between two consecutive segments (from proximal to immediately distal segment).

15. ABIs returning to resting values more than 10 minutes postexercise are a good indication of _____.

16. Independently of the increasing discussion about the "correct" nomenclature to be used to describe continuous wave (CW) Doppler waveforms, a normal CW Doppler waveform from an artery of the lower extremity should be _____.

17. The typical cuff inflation for segmental pulse volume recording (PVR) is _____.

18. CW Doppler and PVR waveforms analysis are examples of _____ criteria for the diagnosis of arterial disease.

19. A normal TBI (toe/brachial index) should be at least _____.

20. Testing for increased sensitivity to cold using immersion in ice water should only be used in patients with suspected _____.

SHORT ANSWER

1. Intermittent claudication and therefore arterial etiology can be easily differentiated from other causes of pain because of what two symptoms?

2. What was the earliest indirect technique used to estimate arterial insufficiency in the lower extremities?

3. For the correct interpretation of results when recording systolic blood pressure, what does the data obtained correspond to?

4. Why is normal resting systolic pressure higher at the ankle than at the brachial (without technical errors)?

5. What are the typical contraindications to exercise in determining the severity of arterial insufficiency in a patient with a relatively normal test at rest?

IMAGE EVALUATION/PATHOLOGY

Review the images and answer the following questions.

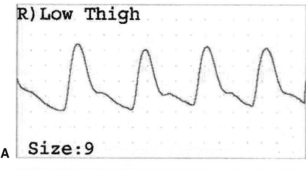

A Size:9

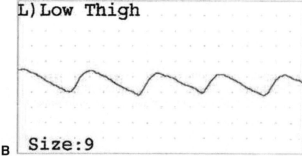

B Size:9

1. These waveforms were most likely obtained using what technique?

2. The "size" (noted as size "9" here) relates to what?

3. Based solely on these images, where would you suspect the primary lesion is?

CASE STUDY

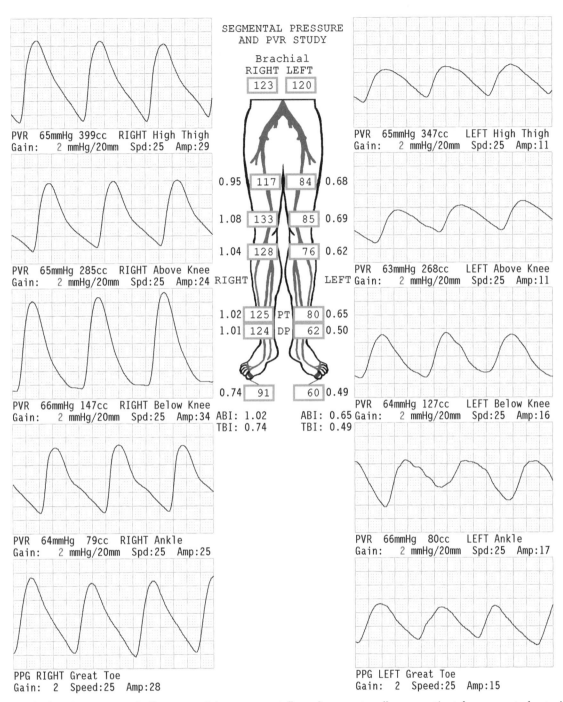

SEGMENTAL PRESSURE
AND PVR STUDY

Brachial
RIGHT LEFT
123   120

PVR 65mmHg 399cc RIGHT High Thigh
Gain: 2 mmHg/20mm Spd:25 Amp:29

PVR 65mmHg 347cc LEFT High Thigh
Gain: 2 mmHg/20mm Spd:25 Amp:11

0.95 117   84 0.68

1.08 133   85 0.69

1.04 128   76 0.62

PVR 65mmHg 285cc RIGHT Above Knee
Gain: 2 mmHg/20mm Spd:25 Amp:24

PVR 63mmHg 268cc LEFT Above Knee
Gain: 2 mmHg/20mm Spd:25 Amp:11

RIGHT   LEFT

1.02 125 PT   80 0.65
1.01 124 DP   62 0.50

PVR 66mmHg 147cc RIGHT Below Knee
Gain: 2 mmHg/20mm Spd:25 Amp:34

0.74 91   60 0.49

ABI: 1.02   ABI: 0.65
TBI: 0.74   TBI: 0.49

PVR 64mmHg 127cc LEFT Below Knee
Gain: 2 mmHg/20mm Spd:25 Amp:16

PVR 64mmHg 79cc RIGHT Ankle
Gain: 2 mmHg/20mm Spd:25 Amp:25

PVR 66mmHg 80cc LEFT Ankle
Gain: 2 mmHg/20mm Spd:25 Amp:17

PPG RIGHT Great Toe
Gain: 2 Speed:25 Amp:28

PPG LEFT Great Toe
Gain: 2 Speed:25 Amp:15

1. You are asked to interpret an indirect arterial assessment (based on protocol) on a patient for suspected arterial insufficiency from one of your staff technologists. The patient is in the intensive care unit and unresponsive at the moment. The patient was recently admitted, and aside from the physician's note stating "decrease pulses" in the left lower extremities, you have no other records available.

The record shows an ABI on the left of 0.65 (at rest!) and the following waveforms as seen on the image. The waveforms are obtained with which technique (explain how you get to this conclusion)? What do the results suggest (based on the analysis of waveforms and ABI)? Were there possibilities of technical errors (explain why or why not)? What other tests could have been performed to add precisions to the diagnosis?

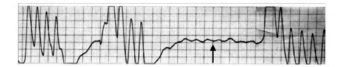

2. A patient is referred to the vascular lab for evaluation for a coronary bypass graft. The patient had several such grafts performed in the past and does not have any more adequate veins. What is an alternate solution for coronary artery grafting? To determine that the vessel chosen will not compromise the arterial circulation of this patient, what is the first and simplest test to perform? If the results of the test show the following (the arrow shows the results with compression of the radial artery), what would you conclude?

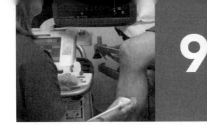

9 Duplex Ultrasound of Lower Extremity Arteries

REVIEW OF GLOSSARY OF TERMS

MATCHING

Match the key terms with their definitions.

Key Terms

1. _____ Duplex arteriography

2. _____ Contrast arteriography

3. _____ Plaque

4. _____ Aneurysm

Definition

a. A radiologic imaging technique performed using ionizing radiation to provide detailed arterial system configuration and pathology information

b. A localized dilation of an artery involving all three layers of the arterial wall

c. Ultrasound imaging of the arterial system performed to identify atherosclerotic disease and other arterial pathology providing a detailed map of the arterial system evaluated

d. The deposit of fatty material within the vessel walls, which is characteristic of atherosclerosis

CHAPTER REVIEW

MULTIPLE CHOICE

1. What is the main technical limitation in the routine use of duplex ultrasound instead of contrast angiography to visualize the arteries of the lower extremities due to?
   a. Most plaque will be calcified
   b. Most equipment does not have that imaging capacity
   c. Most sonographers are not trained to obtain diagnostic data
   d. Most physicians are not trained to interpret data

2. On a posterior approach of the popliteal fossa, what will a large branch identified superior to the popliteal artery most likely be?
   a. The anterior tibial artery
   b. A geniculate artery
   c. A gastrocnemius artery
   d. The tibioperoneal trunk

3. Which artery is best visualized by a posterolateral approach at the level of the calf?
   a. The posterior tibial artery
   b. The peroneal artery
   c. The popliteal artery
   d. The tibioperoneal trunk

4. Which of the following approaches represents good practice to thoroughly evaluate arterial disease in the lower extremities when using B-mode to view the vessel?
   a. In an anterior and posterior approach
   b. In a medial and lateral approach
   c. In a cephalad to caudad approach
   d. In a transverse and longitudinal position

5. What is the primary tool to evaluate disease of the lower extremity arteries using duplex ultrasound (at the exception of aneurysm)?
   a. Aliasing on color Doppler
   b. B-mode image
   c. Color display with power Doppler
   d. Peak systolic velocity

6. How is the velocity ratio (Vr) calculated?
   a. PSV at stenosis divided by PSV proximal to stenosis
   b. PSV proximal to stenosis divided by PSV at stenosis
   c. PSV at stenosis divided by PSV distal to stenosis
   d. PSV distal to stenosis divided by PSV at stenosis

7. Data on which of the following are NOT crucial to best assess for the possibility of treatment of an arterial lesion by an angioplasty or stent (or both)?
   a. Size of the artery
   b. Position of branches
   c. Length of the stenosis
   d. Location of the stenosis

8. Why does duplex ultrasound has an advantage over contrast angiography for the examination of vessel walls?
   a. The plaque thickness can be measured
   b. The plaque characteristics can be determined
   c. The wall thickness can be measured
   d. The remaining lumen can be measured

9. The main pitfall of duplex ultrasound (in general) in examining arterial disease is in the evaluation of which of the following?
   a. Flow at velocities less than 20 cm/s
   b. Flow at velocities over 400 cm/s
   c. Length of occluded segment
   d. Collateral vessels

10. When using duplex ultrasound to record slow flow (<20 cm/s) in an arterial segment, which of the following tools can NOT be used?
    a. Decrease the PRF
    b. Use a low wall filter
    c. Increase the persistence of color
    d. Increase the Doppler gain

11. The appearance of a plaque based on its content is important, but why is characterizing the surface of the plaque also valuable?
    a. Smooth plaque may be more prone to rupture
    b. Smooth plaque is more likely to contain ulcers
    c. Irregular plaque may be more prone to rupture
    d. Irregular plaque may be more stable

12. Why is reporting the presence of a partial thrombus in an aneurysm important?
    a. Partial thrombus may not be visible on contrast angiography
    b. Pieces of thrombus can embolize
    c. The lumen may not be enlarged
    d. It will likely proceed to an acute occlusion

13. When can a greater than 70% stenosis in any arteries of the lower extremities be safely inferred?
    a. The PSV is half distal to the stenosis
    b. The PSV is doubled at the stenosis
    c. The Vr is equal to or greater than 2
    d. The Vr is equal to or greater than 3

14. How is low resistance characterized on Doppler spectrum?
    a. Antegrade flow throughout diastole
    b. Antegrade flow in systole
    c. Retrograde flow is systole
    d. Sharp downstroke in early diastole

15. Which of the following is NOT a potential pathologic finding when the Doppler spectrum of an artery of the lower extremity will display low-resistance characteristics?
    a. Arteriovenous fistula
    b. Postreactive hyperemia
    c. Cellulitis
    d. Trauma

16. Doppler spectra with a characteristic low-resistance outline may be seen distal to a hemodynamically significant stenosis. What will the Doppler spectra also display?
    a. Delay on the downstroke in systole
    b. Delay on the upstroke in systole
    c. Retrograde flow in diastole
    d. Retrograde flow in systole

17. What characteristic outline will Doppler spectra in an arterial segment proximal to a hemodynamically significant stenosis or an occlusion have?
    a. No flow in diastole
    b. No flow in systole
    c. Retrograde flow in diastole
    d. Retrograde flow in systole

18. Which of the following is NOT a factor typically associated with the need to perform a contrast angiography after a limited duplex ultrasound of the arterial system?
    a. High infrapopliteal vessels calcification
    b. Limb-threatening ischemia
    c. Female gender
    d. Older age

19. Why is the use of contrast angiography in diabetic patients particularly worrisome?
    a. Ionizing radiation
    b. Nephrotoxic agents
    c. Poor visualization of calcified segments
    d. Poor visualization of low flow

20. What are the best ultrasound techniques available to determine the hemodynamic significance of an arterial lesion?
    a. Doppler spectrum analysis and color Doppler
    b. Doppler spectrum analysis and flow velocities
    c. Power and color Doppler
    d. Flow velocities and velocity ratio

FILL-IN-THE-BLANK

1. Conditions and risk factors for which patients are referred for duplex ultrasound of the lower extremity arteries are _____ as those for indirect physiologic testing.

2. The below-knee segment of the popliteal artery is best examined through a _____ approach.

3. Most arteries of the lower extremity can be examined by duplex ultrasound using a _____ approach.

4. The two arteries or arterial segments, which cannot be well examined with duplex ultrasound via a medial approach, are the popliteal artery and _____.

5. The superficial femoral artery typically changes name to become the popliteal artery at the following landmark: _____.

6. On a posterior approach of the upper calf, the artery branching off the popliteal artery deep to the popliteal artery is most likely the _____.

7. In general, color and power Doppler's primary advantage is for _____ of the vessels.

8. The degree of stenosis in an artery of the lower extremity is best evaluated by recording PSV and calculating _____.

9. To evaluate the dorsalis pedis artery adequately, a sonographer should be particularly careful with the _____ from the transducer.

10. Duplex ultrasound is superior to contrast angiography in determining a suitable site for a graft distal anastomosis because it can detect _____ area of the vessel wall.

11. Using a lower frequency transducer to view the SFA at Hunter's canal or the tibioperoneal trunk at the upper calf will reduce _____.

12. Determining/characterizing the "nature" of a plaque or even wall thickening is important information a sonographer can convey to a surgeon because _____ through a calcified plaque is almost impossible.

13. Although the PSV (peak systolic velocity) is the primary measurement obtained, stenoses are classified based on _____.

14. Using duplex ultrasound instead of contrast angiography in patients with severe to critical limb ischemia is recommended because the exam with duplex is more _____.

15. Contrast angiography would be contraindicated for patients with severe renal disease because of the use of _____.

16. Very low flow, particularly to assess the patency of possible outflow vessels, is more easily achieved with duplex ultrasound than with contrast angiography with the use of _____.

17. The hemodynamics of arterial lesions/disease is only possible with _____.

18. Factors suggesting that data are unreliable have yet to be identified with CTA and _____.

19. At a measured diameter of 1.1 cm, a common femoral artery would be considered _____.

20. At a measured diameter of 1.1 cm, a popliteal artery would be considered _____.

SHORT ANSWER

1. In evaluation of the arterial tree of the lower extremities with critical limb ischemia, duplex ultrasound is a more useful imaging technique than contrast angiography because it allows accurate visualization of what?

2. A remarkable advantage of duplex ultrasound over other imaging techniques for arterial segment is that the versatility of duplex ultrasound will allow to: (answer)

IMAGE EVALUATION/PATHOLOGY

Review the images and answer the following questions.

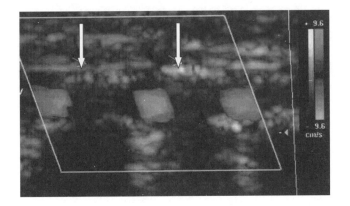

1. What area do the arrows point to?

2. How would you substantiate the answer to the previous question?

3. Is stenosis likely at the area not adequately visualized? Explain.

CASE STUDY

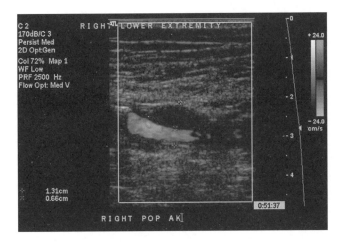

2. A 79-year-old male presents for a consultation in vascular surgery for nonhealing ulcers on several digits of his left foot. On further examination, the patient reveals a history of intermittent claudication: more prominent on the left, the left foot is very cold to the touch, and pulses at the left ankle cannot be felt. Because of the relative emergency of this case presentation, the surgeon elects to send the patient to the vascular lab for examination of the arterial system of the left leg by duplex ultrasound. What are some reasons for the choice (instead of contrast angiography)? What would be areas of particular concerns (to pay particular attention to) with this patient while performing the duplex exam?

1. Based on the above image (Note: the total "lumen" measurement in the most dilated portion is recorded at 1.3 cm), if you obtained this image at the popliteal artery, which pathology would you think of?

What alternative/differential diagnosis could you bring forth (given the location)? How could you confirm the nature of the dilated portion with no color flow?

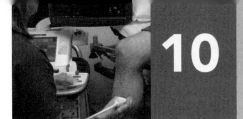

10 Upper Extremity Arterial Duplex Scanning

REVIEW OF GLOSSARY OF TERMS

MATCHING

Match the key terms with their definitions.

Key Terms

1. _____ Thoracic outlet

2. _____ Raynaud's syndrome

3. _____ Takayasu's arteritis

4. _____ Vasospasm

Definition

a. A form of large vessel vasculitis resulting in intimal fibrosis and vessel narrowing

b. A sudden constriction of a blood vessel, which will reduce the lumen and blood flow rate

c. A vasospastic disorder of the digital vessels

d. The superior opening of the thoracic cavity, which is bordered by the clavicle and first rib. The subclavian artery, subclavian vein, and brachial nerve plexus pass through this opening.

ANATOMY AND PHYSIOLOGY REVIEW

IMAGE LABELING

Complete the labels in the image that follows.

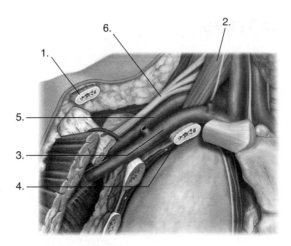

Anatomy of the thoracic outlet.

CHAPTER REVIEW

MULTIPLE CHOICE

1. What percentage of extremity peripheral arterial disease do upper extremities arterial diseases represent?
   a. 5%
   b. 15%
   c. 20%
   d. 50%

2. Which of the following is NOT a prominent etiology of arterial diseases in the upper extremities (arms and forearms)?
   a. Mechanical obstruction or compression at the thoracic outlet
   b. Embolism from various sources (including the heart)
   c. Vasoconstriction of digital arteries
   d. Diffuse atherosclerosis of the axillary or brachial artery

3. What is a dilated segment of the proximal descending aorta (which may give rise to the takeoff of an aberrant subclavian artery) known as?
   a. Ortner syndrome
   b. Thoracic outlet syndrome
   c. Raynaud's syndrome
   d. Kommerell diverticulum

4. Which of the following can NOT cause compression of the subclavian artery?
   a. Compression between the first rib and scalene muscle
   b. Compression between the clavicle and first rib
   c. Compression by brachial plexus
   d. Compression by the pectoralis minor

5. Which of the following is NOT a potential consequence of compression of the subclavian artery at the thoracic outlet?
   a. Thrombosis
   b. Embolism
   c. Stenosis
   d. Aneurysm

6. Injury of what artery may result in hypothenar hammer syndrome?
   a. The radial artery at the wrist
   b. The interosseous artery at the wrist
   c. The ulnar artery at the wrist
   d. The posterior branch of the radial artery

7. The sternal notch window, the infraclavicular, and supraclavicular approaches are all used to visualize the origin of which of the following?
   a. The subclavian arteries
   b. The innominate arteries
   c. The common carotid arteries
   d. The axillary arteries

8. Under normal conditions, flow velocities range of 40 to 60 cm/s are typical for:
   a. Large feeding arteries to the upper extremities
   b. Arteries in the forearm
   c. Arteries in the arm
   d. All arteries in the upper extremities

9. What did one study find that over 40% of aneurysms of the subclavian arteries were associated with?
   a. Vasospasm
   b. Injury or trauma
   c. Thoracic outlet syndrome
   d. Raynaud's disease

10. Aside from the subclavian artery, which artery may be prone to aneurysms (under particular circumstances) in the upper extremities?
    a. The radial artery
    b. The ulnar artery
    c. The brachial artery
    d. The axillary artery

11. How is primary Raynaud's syndrome distinguished from secondary Raynaud's syndrome or Raynaud's phenomenon?
    a. There are underlying diseases
    b. There are no underlying diseases
    c. There is no distinction
    d. The symptoms are different

12. Although rare, digital arteries occlusion from embolization may occur. Which of the following is NOT a predominant source of embolization?
    a. Subclavian artery aneurysms
    b. Stenosis of proximal upper extremity arteries
    c. Fibromuscular diseases of arteries of the forearm
    d. Atrial fibrillation

13. To efficiently assess perfusion and/or vasospasm of digital arteries, how should one record waveforms obtained with PPG?
    a. Pre- and postwarming of fingers
    b. Pre- and postexercise
    c. Pre- and postcold immersion
    d. Pre- and postarm abduction

14. Compression of structures at the thoracic outlet may happen with all of the following EXCEPT:
    a. Hypertrophy of the scalene muscle
    b. Hypertrophy of the pectoralis minor muscle
    c. Presence of a cervical rib
    d. Presence of abnormal fibrous bands

15. Which of the following statements regarding compression of the brachial plexus and vascular structures at the thoracic outlet is FALSE?
    a. Compression of either will give similar symptoms
    b. Compression of either cannot be easily confirmed by provocative maneuvers
    c. Compression of both often occurs concomitantly
    d. Confirmation of neural symptoms is best done by electromyography (EMG)

16. How is "arterial minor" form of thoracic outlet syndrome defined?
    a. Intermittent compression of the subclavian artery when arm is in neutral position
    b. Significant compression of the subclavian artery by clavicle
    c. Intermittent compression of the subclavian when arm is raised overhead
    d. Significant compression of the subclavian artery by first rib

17. Which of the following conditions is associated with significant stenosis or occlusion of arteries of the arm and/or forearm from atherosclerosis?
    a. Diabetes and/or renal failure
    b. Coronary artery disease
    c. Peripheral arterial disease
    d. Systemic diseases

18. In a patient on hemodialysis presenting with digital ischemia and gangrene, what is the most likely etiology?
    a. Steal phenomenon from the dialysis access
    b. Buerger's disease
    c. Raynaud's syndrome
    d. Arterial disease linked to end-stage renal disease

19. Which form of arterial inflammation can affect the ophthalmic artery as well as the subclavian or axillary?
    a. Takayasu's
    b. Raynaud's
    c. Buerger's
    d. Giant cell arteritis

20. What is the most significant difference between giant cell arteritis and Takayasu's disease when both affect the subclavian artery?
    a. The age of the patient
    b. The gender of the patient
    c. The health of the patient
    d. The body habitus of the patient

FILL-IN-THE-BLANK

1. The vertebral arteries are the first major branches of _____.

2. This vertebral artery arises in 4% to 6% directly from the aortic arch, on the _____.

3. The artery resting between the biceps muscle anteriorly and triceps muscle posteriorly is _____.

4. The artery, which lies deep to the pectoralis major and minor, is _____.

5. High takeoff may occur as a variant of the radial artery but also _____.

6. The interosseous artery commonly takes off from _____.

7. The pledge position of the arm is the most efficient position to examine the _____ by duplex.

8. Using the sternal notch window, the origin of the subclavian artery is usually first indentified with color Doppler in a _____ view.

9. With Doppler, all arteries in the upper extremities should, under normal conditions, exhibit _____.

10. To assist in the visualization of the relatively small caliber arteries in the forearm, the sonographer may use _____ of the arm.

11. Secondary Raynaud's syndrome is often seen with _____.

12. Aside from scleroderma, secondary Raynaud's syndrome may be seen with this other systemic disease: _____.

13. Digital arteries necrosis associated with Raynaud's symptoms will rarely be seen with _____.

14. The most efficient technique to assess vasospasm of digital arteries and therefore perfusion of these arteries is _____.

15. Provocative maneuvers demonstrating subclavian artery stenosis at the thoracic outlet may occur in 20% of _____ individuals.

16. Unilateral digital ischemia should prompt the sonographer to look for a source of _____ from more proximal arteries.

17. Clinically significant stenosis or occlusion of upper extremity arteries from atherosclerosis is typically confined to _____.

18. Symptoms of fever, malaise, arthralgia, and myalgia are not uncommon in the _____ phase of Takayasu's disease.

19. Immunosuppressant and anti-inflammatory medications are the primary treatment for several forms of _____.

20. A definite diagnosis for Buerger's disease is best achieved with _____.

SHORT ANSWER

1. What is a retroesophageal subclavian artery?

2. The terminal branches of the radial artery anastomose with both what?

3. The vertebral arteries are distinguished from the thyrocervical and costocervical trunks by the profile of the Doppler spectrum with the vertebral arteries displaying what?

4. From epidemiologic studies, it was found that the two most reliable criteria, correlating with >50% stenosis in an upper extremity artery, were:

5. After traumatic injuries to the upper extremities, examination by duplex ultrasound should focus on evaluating for:

IMAGE EVALUATION/PATHOLOGY

Review the images and answer the following questions.

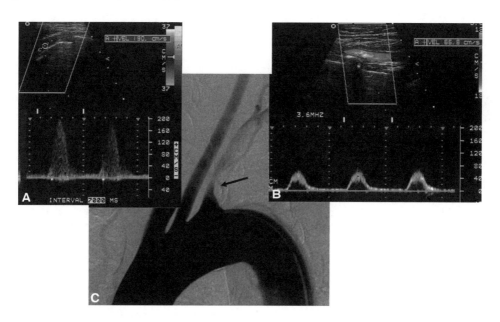

1. Which of the Doppler spectrums (A) or (B) would best represent what could be expected at the area designated by the arrow on angiogram (C)?

2. Which artery is showing pathology?

3. Where could you find Doppler spectrum (B)? Distal or proximal to the stenosis?

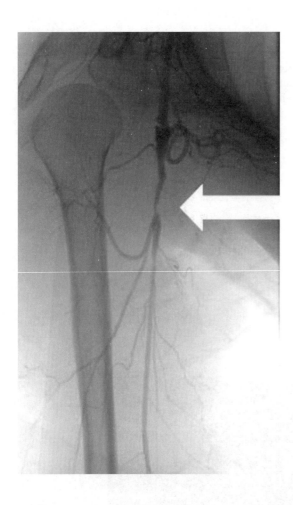

4. Based on the landmarks visible on this angiogram, the arrow points to a defect in which vessel?

5. What would you expect to see with corresponding Doppler and color Doppler on ultrasound?

CASE STUDY

1. A healthy 45-year-old female presents to the vascular lab (located in Vermont) in mid-February, with ischemic changes in both thumbs and several digits of her feet. What should your questions focus on? What should probably be the first exam? She reveals that she is an avid skier and spends most of her free time "on the slopes." What do you expect the results of first exam to reveal?

2. A 25-year-old male working for the civil engineering department of the city presents with a pulsatile mass on the level of the lateral aspect of the wrist extending slightly to the upper palm of his right hand. Small ischemic changes are also evident at the tip of the fourth and fifth fingers. What is the most probable cause for this presentation of signs? What is the best test you could use for diagnosis in the vascular lab? What do you expect the most likely results will reveal?

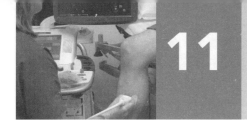

REVIEW OF GLOSSARY OF TERMS

MATCHING

Match the key terms with their definitions.

Key Terms

1. _____ Bypass
2. _____ Graft
3. _____ In situ bypass
4. _____ Anastomosis
5. _____ Arteriovenous fistula
6. _____ Hyperemia

Definitions

a. A conduit that can be prosthetic material or autogenous vein used to divert blood flow from one artery to another
b. A connection between an artery and vein that was created as a result of surgery or by other iatrogenic means
c. A channel that diverts blood flow from one artery to another, usually done to shunt flow around an occluded portion of a vessel
d. The great saphenous vein is left in place in its normal anatomical position and used to create a diversionary channel for blood flow around an occluded artery
e. An increase in blood flow. This can occur following exercise. It can also occur following restoration of blood flow following periods of ischemia.
f. A connection created surgically to connect two vessels that were formerly not connected

ANATOMY AND PHYSIOLOGY REVIEW

IMAGE LABELING

Complete the labels in the images that follow.

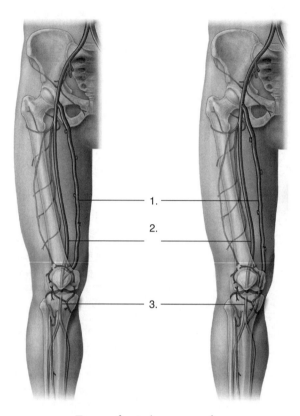

Types of vein bypass grafts.

CHAPTER REVIEW

MULTIPLE CHOICE

1. Of the following, which is NOT considered a method of assessment of a lower extremity infrainguinal bypass graft?
   a. Physical/clinical evaluation
   b. Ankle to brachial index
   c. Chemical blood chemistry panel
   d. Plethysmography

2. Which of the following veins would be typically used for an in situ bypass in the lower extremity?
   a. The cephalic vein
   b. The basilic vein
   c. The small saphenous vein
   d. The great saphenous vein

3. Which of the following issues with synthetic grafts is NOT a potential risk for failure of the graft?
   a. High thrombogenic potential
   b. High rate of technical problems
   c. High rate of progressive stenosis at the inflow artery
   d. High rate of progressive stenosis at the outflow artery

4. Why are in situ infrainguinal bypass grafts using the great saphenous vein a common and preferred technique?
   a. There is a better match of vessel size at the inflow and outflow
   b. There is no need to lyze the valves
   c. The branches of the great saphenous vein provide additional collateral
   d. This allows for reverse flow

5. What is the term to describe an autogenous vein graft where the vein retains its original anatomical direction?
   a. Reverse
   b. In situ
   c. Orthograde
   d. Retrograde

6. Independently of the type of bypass grafts used, where is the distal anastomosis typically located?
   a. Distal to the disease
   b. Proximal to the disease
   c. At the level of the popliteal artery
   d. At the level of the dorsalis pedis

7. Which of the following is NOT one of the main causes for early autogenous vein graft thrombosis (within the first 30 days)?
   a. Underlying hypercoagulable state
   b. Entrapment of the graft
   c. Inadequate vein conduit
   d. Inadequate run-off bed

8. Which amount of gray scale images, spectral Doppler, and color Doppler describes the minimum suggested documentation for evaluation of a bypass graft?
   a. Inflow and outflow only with additional ABI
   b. Inflow and outflow only with additional PVR
   c. Inflow and outflow, proximal and distal anastomosis, mid-graft
   d. Proximal and distal anastomoses only

9. When a stenosis is detected in the postoperative evaluation of a bypass graft, what should the spectral Doppler be used to record?
   a. PSV only
   b. EDV only
   c. PSV ratio
   d. PSV and EDV

10. Which of the following arteries is NOT commonly used as inflow for a bypass graft in the lower extremities?
    a. Common femoral artery
    b. Profunda femoris
    c. Geniculate artery
    d. Popliteal artery

11. Which of the following arteries is NOT commonly used as outflow for a bypass graft in the lower extremities?
    a. The popliteal artery
    b. The dorsalis pedis artery
    c. The posterior tibial artery
    d. The proximal superficial femoral artery

12. Which of the following may require a more aggressive surveillance program (every 2 months or less) for a bypass graft?
    a. A Dacron graft
    b. A PTFE graft
    c. A graft that has undergone revision or thrombectomy
    d. A graft where the distal anastomosis in the dorsalis pedis artery

13. Which of the following is NOT a potential incidental finding related to the perigraft space?
    a. Venous thrombosis
    b. Seroma
    c. Hematoma
    d. Abscesses

14. Where will myointimal hyperplasia in an autogenous vein graft typically occur?
    a. At the proximal anastomosis
    b. At the distal anastomosis
    c. At a site of previous valve sinus
    d. In the mid-graft only

15. What are intimal flaps or dissection, which occasionally occur in bypass grafts, typically the result of?
    a. Valve retention
    b. Intraoperative technical problem
    c. Fibrosis in the inflow artery
    d. Aneurysms at the distal anastomosis

16. In synthetic aortofemoral or femoro-femoral grafts, where may pseudoaneurysms, while rare, occur?
    a. The mid-graft
    b. Anywhere along the length of the graft
    c. The distal anastomosis
    d. The femoral anastomosis

17. Arteriovenous fistula, occasionally seen in in situ bypass grafts, results from failure to ligate which of the following?
    a. The small saphenous vein
    b. A perforating vein
    c. A small arterial branch
    d. A defect at valve lysis

18. How is mean graft velocity assessed?
    a. Taking several measurements at the mid-graft level
    b. Averaging the velocities at the proximal and distal anastomoses
    c. Averaging the velocities from the inflow and outflow arteries
    d. Averaging three or four velocities from nonstenotic segment

19. What is the first data source that should be used to examine a bypass graft?
    a. B-mode
    b. Spectral Doppler
    c. Color Doppler
    d. Power Doppler

20. On follow-up of a bypass graft done 4 years ago, what may a Doppler spectrum displaying delay in systole indicate?
    a. Defect at the anastomosis
    b. Progression of disease at the inflow
    c. Arteriovenous fistula within the graft
    d. Imminent failure from distal occlusion

FILL-IN-THE-BLANK

1. Duplex ultrasound has been shown to be reliable in the detection of significant pathology in infrainguinal bypass graft in _____ patients.

2. Combining physiologic study with duplex ultrasound for the assessment of an infrainguinal bypass graft is important for the detection of significant pathology and the evaluation of _____.

3. Types of bypass grafts can be categorized based on the material used for the graft and _____.

4. Vein grafts have a longer patency rate than synthetic grafts (independently of the location) because vein grafts are less _____.

5. Types of materials used for infrainguinal bypass grafts include autogenous veins, synthetic materials, and _____.

6. Within the first 30 days of the perioperative period following the implantation of a bypass graft, the most common problems are _____.

7. In the postoperative period, 75% of graft revisions are done for stenoses at the _____.

8. Spectral Doppler documentation for the evaluation of a bypass graft is done to acquire data on _____.

9. To document a stenosis within a bypass graft most completely, the PSV and EDV proximal, within, and distal to the stenosis should be noted, as well as _____.

10. To ensure accurate documentation during a follow-up for a bypass graft, it is important for the sonographer to be familiar with the type and location of the bypass, and therefore refer to _____.

11. Twenty-four months after a bypass graft has been performed, the main cause of failure will be _____.

12. The issue referred to in question 11 will affect in particular _____.

13. During follow-up exams of bypass graft using comparison of flow velocities for diagnostic purpose, an effort should be made to obtain the velocities in the same location, as well as with the same _____.

14. Color Doppler can be useful in the evaluation of a bypass for defects can be seen because of _____.

15. Although located in the lower extremities, Doppler spectrum in a bypass graft can typically display _____-resistance characteristics.

16. A complication unique to in situ bypass graft is _____.

17. A decrease of mean graft flow velocity of more than _____ from previous exam is indicative of potential failure of the graft.

18. To thoroughly examine the presence of retained valve and/or intimal flap, it is recommended to turn off _____.

19. A tunneled PTFE femoral to popliteal graft will be _____ than an in situ graft.

20. To examine the distal anastomosis and outflow of a femoral to dorsalis pedis bypass graft, one may opt to select a transducer with _____ frequency.

SHORT ANSWER

1. What is an important feature when choosing autogenous veins for infrainguinal bypass grafts in a reverse position?

2. What are the typical causes of graft failures more than 24 months after implantation?

IMAGE EVALUATION/PATHOLOGY

Review the images and answer the following questions.

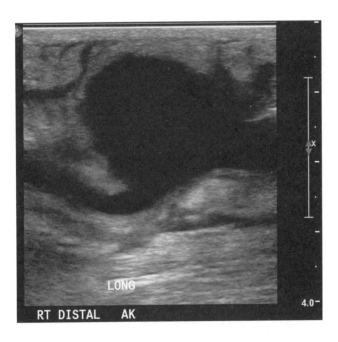

1. What pathology can be seen in the figure?

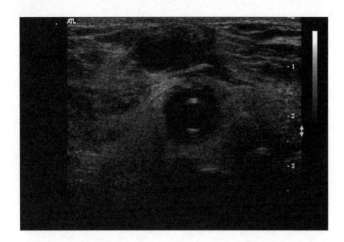

2. What does this image suggest?

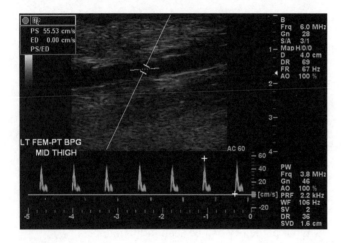

3. What does the Doppler waveform pattern seen in this image seem to suggest?

CASE STUDY

1. A 75-year-old male with long-standing history of cardiovascular diseases and vascular reconstruction in the lower extremities presents with a pulsatile mass in the left inguinal area. The history of vascular reconstruction includes an aortobifemoral bypass graft and a right femoral to popliteal bypass graft. The patient is now postcardiac catheterization. What would you suspect the pulsatile mass to be? What other scenario could you suggest based on the history?

2. An 81-year-old female presents to the vascular lab with a cold right foot and evidence of ulceration on several digits of the right foot. She is not one of your regular patients. You do not have any records on this patient and she cannot recall what was done or when, but you see some scars on the medial aspect of the leg, suggesting that a bypass graft may have been done. What should you assess first?

You decide to use duplex ultrasound to get an idea of what was done. Slightly below the inguinal ligament, you see the takeoff of a "vessel" with bright white line and flow with spectral and color Doppler. What does this finding suggest?

You cannot assess the graft further than 1 to 2 cm distal to the anastomosis, so you sample the proximal portion of the graft and attempt to find the distal anastomosis or outflow. You obtain a Doppler signal at the popliteal artery. The Doppler spectrum in the proximal graft shows PSV of 130 cm/s with no diastolic flow and very sharp but narrow waveforms. The Doppler spectrum at the popliteal artery shows delay in systole and a PSV of 11 cm/s with diastolic flow. What can you infer from these data?

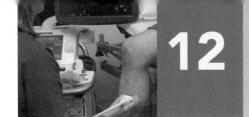

12 Ultrasound Following Interventional Procedures

REVIEW OF GLOSSARY OF TERMS

MATCHING

Match the key terms with their definitions.

Key Terms

1. _____ Angioplasty

2. _____ Atherectomy

3. _____ Dissection

4. _____ Hyperplasia

5. _____ Stent

Definition

a. A tear along the inner layer of an artery that results in the splitting or separation of the walls of a blood vessel

b. A tubelike structure placed inside a blood vessel to provide patency and support

c. A nonsurgical procedure to remove plaque from an artery using a special catheter with a device at the tip that cuts away the plaque

d. An abnormal increase in the number of cells; myointimal hyperplasia; an increase in the number of smooth muscle cells within the intima in response to vessel injury

e. A surgical repair of a blood vessel by reconstructing or replacing part of the vessel. The procedure can be done with a balloon-tipped catheter that is used to enlarge a narrowing (stenosis) in a blood vessel.

CHAPTER REVIEW

MULTIPLE CHOICE

1. Which of the following is NOT a consideration for treatment options for vascular diseases of the upper or lower extremities?
   a. The location and extent of disease
   b. The comorbid factors
   c. The etiology of disease
   d. The risk–benefit ratio of the procedure

2. Which of the following is NOT one of the endovascular treatments of choice for more extensive arterial stenosis?
   a. Balloon angioplasty
   b. Subintimal angioplasty
   c. Mechanical atherectomy
   d. Stent graft angioplasty

3. The TASC (Trans-Atlantic Inter-Society Consensus) II offers criteria to plan for interventions for arterials disease based on which of the following?
   a. The type of lesions
   b. The etiology and severity of the disease
   c. The extension and etiology of the disease
   d. The location and severity of the disease

4. Endovascular procedures would be more appropriate for which lesions (TASC II classification)?
   a. TASC A and B lesions
   b. TASC C and D lesions
   c. TASC A and C lesions
   d. TASC B and D lesions

5. Which of the following is NOT associated with poor outcomes (high risk of failure) of endovascular procedures?
   a. Diabetes
   b. Renal failure
   c. Coronary disease
   d. Tibial disease

6. Which of the following is NOT a symptom of poor limb reperfusion postendovascular procedure?
   a. Claudication
   b. Restenosis
   c. Rest pain
   d. Ulcers

7. Relying on patient's history to assess successful reperfusion of a limb is a particular challenge when patients are:
   a. Active
   b. Sedentary
   c. Diabetic
   d. Obese

8. Which of the following is NOT part of the referral documentation for exams in the vascular lab following an endovascular procedure?
   a. Indications for the referral
   b. Type of intervention performed
   c. Risk factors for underlying disease
   d. Location of the intervention performed

9. The prevalence of restenosis after endovascular procedure in the femoropopliteal segment of the arterial tree is highest with which procedure?
   a. Balloon angioplasty
   b. Stent graft
   c. Atherectomy
   d. Angioplasty

10. Which of the following is NOT a new "abnormal" finding after an endovascular procedure?
    a. A 50% stenosis or more proximal to the treated area
    b. A 50% stenosis or more within the treated area
    c. A 50% stenosis or more distal to the treated area
    d. All of the above

11. Several studies have shown a good correlation between stenosis of 70% or more at the site of previous endovascular procedures with which of the following?
    a. Velocities >300 cm/s
    b. Velocity ration of at least 3.5
    c. Both A and B
    d. Neither A nor B

12. Why are flow velocities in a stent (without evidence of restenosis) usually increased compared to velocities in a native artery?
    a. A stent decreases the compliance of the arterial wall
    b. A stent increases the compliance of the arterial wall
    c. A stent decreases the resistance of the tissue
    d. A stent increases the resistance of the tissue

FILL-IN-THE-BLANK

1. The most common endovascular procedure to address an arterial stenosis is _____.

2. Focal endovascular interventions may not restore peripheral pulse because atherosclerosis is usually a _____.

3. It has been estimated that approximately _____ of lesions treated with endovascular procedures will require another intervention within the first year.

4. Follow-up or sequential duplex ultrasound exams are recommended after an endovascular procedure because atherosclerotic lesions often _____.

5. A toe pressure of at least _____ is a good predictor of adequate perfusion to heal an ulcer.

6. An ABI value should be at least _____ higher than the pre-intervention ABI to correlate with limb perfusion improvement.

7. Toe pressure below 30 mm Hg is usually synonymous with _____.

8. The most common cause for restenosis independently of the endovascular procedure performed is _____.

9. The functional significance of a stenosis should always be assessed with _____.

10. Severity of stenosis or disease postendovascular procedures is commonly reported in one of _____ categories.

11. A stent fracture can be suspected on duplex ultrasound if _____ is detected.

12. The outcome status following an additional intervention to restore patency postendovascular procedure is referred to as _____.

IMAGE EVALUATION/PATHOLOGY

Review the images and answer the following questions.

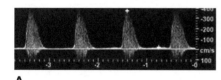 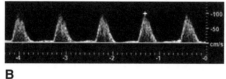 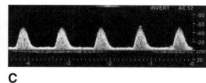

A   B   C

1. Which Doppler spectrum is most likely to be taken proximal to a stenosis?

2. Which Doppler spectrum is most likely to be taken at a stenosis?

3. Which Doppler spectrum is most likely to be taken distal to a stenosis?

4. The velocities seen on Doppler spectrum are consistent with what?

CASE STUDY

1. A 63-year-old female treated for a focal external iliac artery lesion with balloon angioplasty and stent graft presents for a 6-month follow-up in the vascular lab. On assessing the stented area, you keep in mind that in this period of time, the most likely "failure" would involve what?

    On duplex ultrasound examination you find PSV within the stented area of 150 cm/s and a PSV ratio of 2.0, what would you conclude?

    The patient describes symptoms of calf claudication, and the ABI reveals a drop of 0.2 (at rest) from the pre-procedure value. What would you conclude?

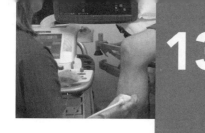

13 Special Considerations in Evaluating Nonatherosclerotic Arterial Pathology

REVIEW OF GLOSSARY OF TERMS

MATCHING

Match the key terms with their definitions.

Key Terms

1. _____ Vascular arteritis
2. _____ Giant cell arteritis
3. _____ Buerger's disease
4. _____ Takayasu's arteritis
5. _____ Embolism
6. _____ Aneurysm
7. _____ Pseudoaneurysm
8. _____ Arteriovenous fistula

Definition

a. An obstruction or occlusion of a blood vessel by a transported clot of blood, mass, bacteria, or other foreign substance
b. An inflammatory disease that affects the blood vessels
c. A type of vascular arteritis that affects the aortic arch and its large branches
d. A type of vascular arteritis also known as thromboangitis obliterans; it affects small and medium-sized arteries
e. A type of vascular arteritis also known as temporal arteritis, which is associated with the superficial temporal artery and other arteries of the head and neck
f. An abnormal communication between an artery and vein, which can be the result of iatrogenic injury or trauma or may be congenitally acquired
g. A dilation of an artery wall involving all three layers of the vessel wall
h. An expanding hematoma; a hole in the arterial wall that allows blood to leave the vessel and collect in the surrounding tissue

CHAPTER REVIEW

MULTIPLE CHOICE

1. Of the following, which could be classified as an acquired disease of an artery?
   a. Occlusion of the distal digital arteries by embolism
   b. Thrombosis of the common femoral artery
   c. An iatrogenic arteriovenous fistula
   d. An aneurysm of the popliteal artery

2. The inflammatory process encountered with most arteritis involve fibrosis of which of the following?
   a. The media layer of the arterial wall
   b. The intima layer of the arterial
   c. The adventitia layer of the arterial wall
   d. None of the layers of the arterial wall

3. Although the exact etiology of most forms of arteritis is unknown, what is it believed that most forms involve?
   a. An immune reaction
   b. An inflammatory process
   c. A fibrosis of the vessel wall
   d. Thrombosis of the vessel lumen

4. In a patient presenting with asymmetrical blood pressures AND no evidence of stenosis of the subclavian artery, what should one suspect?
   a. Buerger's disease
   b. Takayasu's disease
   c. Vasospasm of the axillary artery
   d. Pseudoaneurysm of the brachial artery

5. In a patient presenting with signs and symptoms of giant cell arteritis and asymmetrical blood pressures, what should also be assessed?
   a. The aortic arch
   b. The lower extremity arteries
   c. The upper extremity arteries
   d. The digits

6. What does Takayasu's arteritis mostly affect?
   a. The common carotid arteries
   b. The innominate artery
   c. The axillary arteries
   d. The subclavian arteries

7. What is the best tool available with duplex ultrasound to distinguish arteritis from atherosclerosis diseases?
   a. B-mode
   b. Doppler spectrum
   c. Color Doppler
   d. Power Doppler

8. When present, where will lower extremity claudication symptoms with thromboangitis obliterans most likely be localized?
   a. The arch of the foot
   b. The ankle
   c. The calf
   d. The thigh

9. Digital ischemia can be seen with many different conditions. When would thromboangitis obliterans be suspected as the etiology of the ischemia?
   a. The disease only affect the digits of the feet
   b. The disease only affect the digits of the hands
   c. The disease in present in the digits of one limb and not the other
   d. The disease is present bilaterally

10. What is it necessary to evaluate to obtain a proper diagnosis of Buerger's disease?
    a. Ankle or wrist with Doppler
    b. Proximal large arteries with duplex
    c. Indirect testing with PVR
    d. Digits with PPG

11. Although radiation-induced arteritis lesions often resemble atherosclerotic lesions, the distinction can be made because the lesions with atherosclerosis will be:
    a. Localized
    b. Widespread
    c. Necrotic
    d. Highly calcified

12. A cardiac source of arterial embolism can be seen with all the following EXCEPT:
    a. Atrial fibrillation
    b. Endocarditis
    c. Ventricular septal defect
    d. Left ventricle thrombus

13. Pseudoaneurysms can be seen with all of the following EXCEPT:
    a. Postcardiac catheterization
    b. As inflammatory response
    c. At site of infection of synthetic grafts
    d. With dialysis access grafts

14. What has the "Yin-Yang" symbol been used to describe?
    a. The flow pattern in an arteriovenous fistula
    b. The flow pattern in an aneurysm sac
    c. The flow pattern at an area of dissection
    d. The flow pattern in a pseudoaneurysm sac

15. What are most iatrogenic arteriovenous fistula the result of?
    a. Femoral catheterization
    b. Central venous line placement
    c. Penetrating wounds
    d. Total knee replacement

16. Which of the following statements about popliteal entrapment syndrome is FALSE?
    a. It affects males predominantly
    b. It affect both limbs predominantly
    c. It is an acquired condition
    d. It is a congenital condition

17. What is the preferred maneuver to diagnose popliteal entrapment syndrome?
    a. Walking
    b. Active plantar flexion
    c. Rotating limb
    d. Elevating limb

18. Which of the following conditions is a congenital disorder of connective tissue often resulting in aneurysm formation?
    a. Buerger's
    b. Takayasu's
    c. Ehlers-Danlos
    d. Kawasaki

19. Which of the following can be a secondary site for aneurysm development associated with Marfan syndrome?
    a. The renal artery
    b. The common femoral artery
    c. The posterior tibial artery
    d. The popliteal artery

20. Which of the following is a devastating complication of Ehlers-Danlos syndrome?
    a. Arterial rupture
    b. Aneurysm
    c. Thrombosis
    d. Atherosclerosis

FILL-IN-THE-BLANK

1. The symptoms described by patients suffering from some forms of arteritis are _____ to the symptoms of patients with atherosclerosis.

2. This form of arteritis is rarely seen in patients younger than 50 years old: _____.

3. This form of arteritis is rarely seen in males: _____.

4. Takayasu's disease process, along with the possible occlusion of the vessel lumen, may be complicated by the formation of _____.

5. The appearance of the subclavian artery with Takayasu's disease may involve long stenotic segments followed by _____.

6. This form of inflammatory arterial disease affects males predominantly: _____.

7. Although smoking is always present in the history of patients suffering from Buerger's disease, it is even more prominent in areas where smoking involves _____.

8. This form of arteritis is acquired: _____.

9. Arterial lesions present in radiation-induced arteritis will usually lead to symptoms of claudication _____ after completion of radiation therapy.

10. The symptoms observed with embolic disease are often _____.

11. It has been shown that 80% to 99% of arterial embolisms have a _____ source.

12. Epidemiologic studies have shown that the site outside the cerebral circulation most commonly affected by arterial embolization is _____.

13. Outside the heart, the most common source of arterial emboli is _____.

14. The most common site of iatrogenic pseudoaneurysm is the _____.

15. The characteristic flow pattern observed on a Doppler spectrum at the level of the neck of a pseudoaneurysm is often referred to as _____.

16. A bruit is found on _____, whereas a thrill is found on _____.

17. Arterial closure devices used post-catheterization have occasionally been the cause of _____.

18. One cause of congenital arterial stenosis or occlusion is _____.

19. Behcet syndrome has been associated as a source of nonatherosclerotic _____.

SHORT ANSWER

1. Why can nonatherosclerotic diseases usually be assessed clinically?

2. What causes the hypoechoic wall thickening seen on ultrasound around a temporal artery?

3. Takayasu's disease has been associated as a common source of nonatherosclerotic aneurysms. What is another inflammatory arterial disease that can result in aneurysms?

IMAGE EVALUATION/PATHOLOGY

Review the images and answer the following questions.

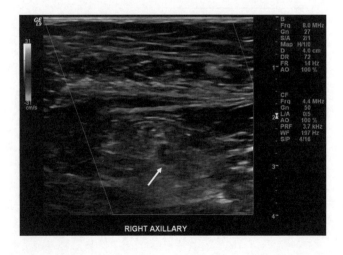

RIGHT AXILLARY

1. The arrow points to the right axillary of a patient. What does the appearance of the lumen and the location of the disease suggest?

2. What is the appearance of the disease in the lumen sometimes called?

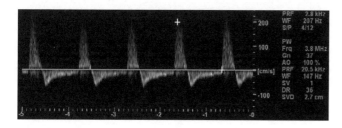

3. What does this Doppler spectrum show?

4. Where can this spectrum typically be observed?

5. What is this spectrum commonly referred to as?

CASE STUDY

1. A 59-year-old male presents to the vascular lab with a pulsatile mass at the level of the dorsal aspect of the right ankle. This unusual presentation puzzles you for a while because you lack documentation of medical history on this patient. You proceed with obtaining a history and a brief physical examination with this patient. What will be the focus of your questions and physical examination?

   You proceed with a duplex ultrasound and obtain a clear image of a mass with flow displaying a "yin-yang" pattern connected by a neck to the distal anterior tibial artery. What rare pathology do you conclude that you found?

2. A 19-year-old female presents to the vascular lab with claudication symptoms at the calf level bilaterally. She is slightly overweight and not very active physically and justifies her condition because of excruciating pain she feels upon walking. She does not have any other relevant risk factors or relevant medical history. Based on her age, symptoms, and history, your first instinct would lead you to focus on which area? Upon examination of the area of focus, you cannot find anything remarkable (no increased velocities), but the spatial relation of the artery and vein does not seem "quite right." What probable cause for her pain do you start thinking of? To confirm your diagnosis, you decide to obtain Doppler spectrum and velocities in the artery with duplex ultrasound while the patient performs which maneuver?

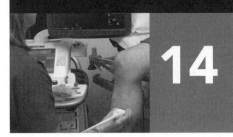

PART 4 • PERIPHERAL VENOUS

14 Duplex Imaging of the Lower Extremity Venous System

REVIEW OF GLOSSARY OF TERMS

MATCHING

Match the key terms with their definitions.

Key Terms

1. _____ Deep vein
2. _____ Superficial vein
3. _____ Perforating vein
4. _____ Acute thrombus
5. _____ Chronic thrombus
6. _____ Valve

Definition

a. Newly formed clotted blood within a vein, generally less than 14 days old
b. A vein that is the companion vessel to an artery and travels within the deep muscular compartments of the leg
c. An inward projection of the intimal layer of a vein wall producing two semilunar leaflets, which present the retrograde movement of blood flow
d. A small vein that connects the deep and superficial venous systems; a vein that passes between the deep and superficial compartments of the leg
e. Clotted blood within a vein that has generally been present for a period of several weeks or months
f. A vein that is superior to the muscular compartments of the leg; travels within superficial fascial compartments; has no corresponding companion artery

CHAPTER REVIEW

MULTIPLE CHOICE

1. Which of the following does imaging the lower extremities venous system with ultrasound NOT allow?
   a. Diagnose thrombosis
   b. Determine the age of the thrombus
   c. Determine the source of a pulmonary embolus
   d. Follow up the progression of disease or resolution of thrombus

2. Which of the following does a duplex ultrasound of the venous system of the lower extremity NOT attempt to answer?
   a. The absence of thrombus
   b. The risk factors for thrombosis
   c. The competency of the valves
   d. The age of the thrombus

3. What are the veins found in the calf muscles considered to be?
   a. Deep veins
   b. Superficial veins
   c. Muscular veins
   d. Perforators

4. Which deep vein is NOT accompanied by an artery with the same name?
   a. The deep femoral vein
   b. The common femoral vein
   c. The popliteal vein
   d. The femoral vein

5. What is the main function of the superficial venous system under normal conditions?
   a. Provide a collateral pathway for the deep veins
   b. Connect with the deep system through perforating veins
   c. Help regulate the body temperature
   d. Provide a reservoir for blood

6. Why was a common/traditional school of thought that thrombosis of superficial vein was less likely to be the cause of pulmonary embolism?
   a. Superficial veins are not surrounded by muscles
   b. Superficial veins do not thrombose as easily as deep veins
   c. Superficial veins do not connect to the deep veins
   d. Thrombus usually propagate through perforators

7. Under normal conditions, valves in perforating veins ensure that blood moves in which of the following ways?
   a. Dissipate around the perforator
   b. From the superficial to the deep system
   c. From the deep to the superficial system
   d. Stay in the superficial system

8. From epidemiological studies, what is the percentage of patients that develops postthrombotic symptoms?
   a. 10%
   b. 30%
   c. 50%
   d. 90%

9. Which of the following is NOT considered a non-genetic (or hereditary) factor contributing to DVT?
   a. Neoplasm
   b. Use of birth control pill
   c. Orthopedic surgery
   d. Factor V Leiden

10. Which statement of Virchow triad is confirmed by the observation that a venous thrombus often start at valve cusps?
    a. Wall injury is an important contributing factor
    b. Hypercoagulability is an important contributing factor
    c. Stasis is an important contributing factor
    d. All three states are necessary

11. What would a high probability for DVT correspond to on Well's score?
    a. <3 points
    b. >2 point
    c. >3 points
    d. >5 points

12. When can a false negative D-dimer be seen in the presence of DVT?
    a. The patient has underlying malignancy
    b. The patient has active inflammation/infection
    c. Assay cannot detect high level of fibrin
    d. Assay cannot detect low levels of fibrin

13. For routine operation of a vascular lab, the use of a high-frequency linear transducer (10 to 18 MHz) is NOT recommended for the evaluation of which of the following?
    a. Superficial vein reflux
    b. Perforators
    c. Arm veins
    d. Pediatric patients

14. Why will using a reverse Trendelenburg position to examine the lower extremity venous system make the exam more difficult?
    a. Veins will be collapsed
    b. Veins will be under low pressure
    c. Veins will be deeper
    d. Veins without thrombus will be harder to compress

15. Which of the following is NOT a qualitative Doppler feature evaluated in the venous system?
    a. Continuity of signal
    b. Spontaneity of signal
    c. Phasicity of signal
    d. Augmentation of signal

16. Which of the following large deep veins commonly have a duplicate?
    a. The profunda and popliteal veins
    b. The femoral and popliteal veins
    c. The external iliac and femoral veins
    d. The common femoral and popliteal veins

17. Which veins are one of the major blood reservoirs located in the calf?
    a. The tibial veins
    b. The small saphenous vein
    c. The soleal veins
    d. The gastrocnemius veins

18. What do bright echoes and well-attached thrombus suggest?
    a. Acute thrombosis
    b. Chronic thrombosis
    c. Too much gain
    d. Risks of embolization

19. In what case will indirect assessment of the iliac veins and IVC using Doppler at the common femoral veins suggest no evidence of obstruction?
    a. The Doppler spectrum exhibits phasicity
    b. The Doppler spectrum exhibits pulsatility
    c. The Doppler spectrum exhibits continuity
    d. The Doppler spectrum ceases with Valsalva

20. Which of the following treatment options will expedite the resolution of a thrombus?
    a. Heparin
    b. Coumadin
    c. Thrombectomy
    d. Thrombolysis

FILL-IN-THE-BLANK

1. Duplex ultrasound for the evaluation of the deep and superficial venous system has largely replaced _____ for the detection of DVT.

2. All tibial arteries are accompanied by at least _____.

3. The junction of the great saphenous vein with the common femoral vein usually occurs _____ to the bifurcation of the superficial and deep femoral arteries.

4. The fact that DVT is often undiagnosed or underdiagnosed is probably because DVT is frequently _____.

5. It has been estimated through epidemiological studies that approximately 50% of cases of DVT are _____ diagnosed.

6. The development of venous thrombosis is determined by a balance between clotting factors and _____.

7. Factor V Leiden is considered one of the _____ conditions.

8. Tachypnea, tachycardia, and chest pain are often signs of _____.

9. A palpable cord along the medial aspect of the lower extremity would be a clinical sign for _____.

10. A baker's cyst (or popliteal cyst) would receive _____ points based on Well's scoring of risk factors.

11. The clinical diagnosis of DVT has

_____ sensitivity and specificity.

12. The evaluation of the IVC and iliac veins in most adult patients would require the use of a _____ transducer.

13. The position described as the tilting of the exam table during a venous exam, so that the legs are approximately 20 degrees lower than the upper body, is called _____.

14. The main venous outflow for the calf is the

_____.

15. It is not uncommon for the femoral vein to be

_____.

16. It is not unusual for the _____ vein to share a common trunk with the gastrocnemius vein.

17. The posterior tibial and peroneal veins typically communicate with the _____ veins.

18. Analysis of _____ provides indirect assessment of the iliac vein when evaluated in the common femoral vein.

19. The only way to adequately image the content of the venous lumen to exclude DVT when performing compression is to view the vessel in

_____.

20. Poorly echogenic, poorly attached thrombus in a visibly dilated vein (compare to the artery) suggests _____ thrombosis.

SHORT ANSWER

1. What is it called when the small saphenous vein extends past the popliteal vein and into the thigh?

2. What are Well's criteria?

3. Why is a thrombus in the anterior tibial veins rare?

IMAGE EVALUATION/PATHOLOGY

Review the images and answer the following questions.

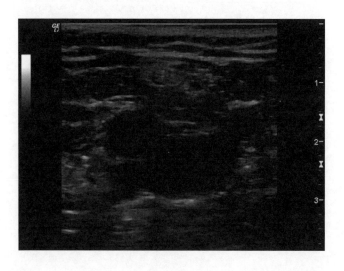

1. The configuration of vessels seen in this image is typically referred to as "Mickey Mouse"; it is usually found in what area of the body?

2. Assuming the transducer is held in a conventional manner, which side of the body was evaluated when this image was taken?

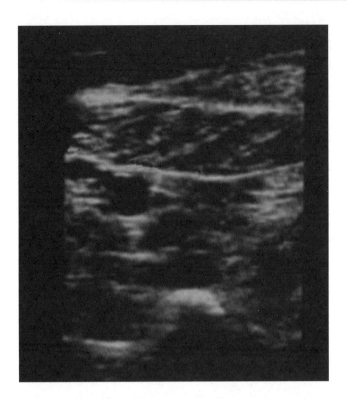

3. What are the vessels represented here?

4. At which level of the lower extremity are you most likely to see this configuration from a medial approach?

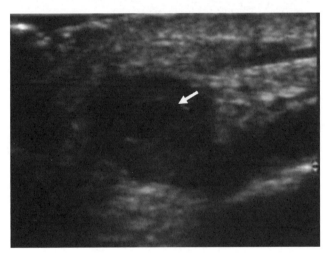

5. What is the arrow pointing at?

6. What does the circumferential area along the vessel wall represent?

7. What was the technique/tool used to allow for visualization in this image?

8. What other techniques/tools could have been used here (for confirming diagnosis)?

CASE STUDY

1. An 86-year-old male presents in the vascular laboratory with a history of right leg edema for 2 weeks. The patient has a history of prostate cancer and IVC filter placement because of previous DVT (diagnosed 1 year ago). The right leg is red and warm from mid-thigh to the ankle. What is probably your first impression? Calculate the Well's score for this patient.

   On duplex examination, you find (right away) a continuous Doppler spectrum at the right and left common femoral veins. Do you revise your first impression? What should you focus on next, given the patient history? What do you expect to find?

2. A 32-year-old female presents in the vascular lab with a history of pain for 3 weeks in the upper to mid-calf on the right leg. She is healthy, athletic, of normal weight, and does not use birth control pills. Calculate the Well's score for this patient.

   The protocol for your lab does not routinely include the evaluation of veins below the knee. Is this a case when an exception is warranted? Why?

   On examination, you find DVT in the peroneal veins. The referring physician orders serial exams and the thrombus appears to propagate toward the popliteal vein. What could you suspect in this case?

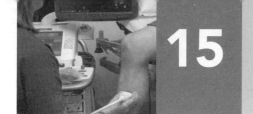

REVIEW OF GLOSSARY OF TERMS

MATCHING

Match the key terms with their definitions.

Key Terms

1. _C_ Valve
2. _d_ Superficial vein
3. _e_ Chronic thrombus
4. _a_ Deep vein
5. _b_ Acute thrombus

Definition

a. A vein that is the companion vessel to an artery and travels within the deep muscular compartments of the leg or arm

b. Newly formed clotted blood within a vein, generally less than 14 days old

c. An inward projection of the intimal layer of a vein wall producing two semilunar leaflets that prevent the retrograde movement of blood flow

d. A vein that is superior to the muscular compartments of the leg or arm; travels within the superficial fascial compartments and has no corresponding companion artery

e. Clotted blood within a vein that has generally been present for a period of several weeks or months

CHAPTER REVIEW

MULTIPLE CHOICE

1. What is the main reason that venous thrombosis in the upper extremities has become more common?
   a. A more sedentary lifestyle
   b. Increased injury to vein walls
   c. An increase in hypercoagulable disease states
   d. Decreased rates of prophylactic anticoagulation

2. Unlike the lower extremities, what do the upper extremities NOT have that may allow spontaneous thrombus formation?
   a. Deep veins
   b. Superficial veins
   c. Soleal sinuses
   d. Respiratory phasic flow dynamics

3. What is venous thrombosis secondary to compression of the subclavian vein at the thoracic inlet known as?
   a. Paget-Schroetter syndrome
   b. May-Thurner syndrome
   c. Raynaud's syndrome
   d. Phlegmasia

4. A patient presents to the vascular lab for upper extremity venous evaluation with face swelling and prominent veins on the chest and neck. What are these symptoms consistent with?
   a. Subclavian vein thrombosis
   b. Cephalic vein thrombosis
   c. Internal jugular vein thrombosis
   d. Superior vena cava thrombosis

5. Transducer compressions are limited over several veins in the upper extremity due to limited access from bony structures. What are the most common veins that are NOT able to be compressed?
   a. Brachiocephalic and subclavian veins
   b. Subclavian and axillary veins
   c. Cephalic and basilic veins
   d. Brachial and radial veins

6. What is the most appropriate transducer for mapping of the upper extremity superficial venous system?
   a. 5 to 10 MHz straight linear array
   b. 5 to 10 MHz curved linear array
   c. 10 to 18 MHz straight linear array
   d. 3.5 to 5 MHz curved linear or sector array

7. The subclavian and jugular veins should be assessed with the patient lying flat to reduce the impact of which of the following?
   a. Hydrostatic pressure
   b. Compression from the clavicle
   c. Heart pulsatility
   d. Respiration

8. The external jugular vein lies _____ to the internal jugular vein.
   a. Anterior
   b. Superior
   c. Deep
   d. Posterior

9. The brachial vein becomes the axillary vein at the confluence with which vein?
   a. Cephalic vein
   b. Radial vein
   c. Basilic vein
   d. Median cubital vein

10. What will taking a quick, deep breath through pursed lips cause the subclavian vein to do, demonstrating coaptation of vein walls?
    a. Dilate
    b. Thrombose
    c. Collapse
    d. Become pulsatile

11. In the upper extremity, in general, which venous system is larger?
    a. Deep system
    b. Superficial system
    c. Deep and superficial are of equal size
    d. Perforating system

12. During upper extremity venous duplex examination, the technologist notes significant pulsatility in the spectral Doppler waveform from the internal jugular vein. What does this finding suggest?
    a. Proximal venous obstruction
    b. Distal venous obstruction
    c. Normal findings for the IJV
    d. Superficial venous obstruction

13. Which of the following vessels may not be routinely evaluated in an UE venous duplex examination but is often added in the event of significant thrombosis?
    a. Internal jugular vein
    b. Subclavian vein
    c. Basilic vein
    d. External jugular vein

14. Because of the location of the brachiocephalic veins, documentation of patency of these vessels is usually performed with which of the following?
    a. Grayscale image with additional color flow and spectral Doppler images
    b. Grayscale imaging alone
    c. Grayscale image with and without transducer compression
    d. Color flow imaging alone

15. What connects the basilic and cephalic veins?
    a. Radial veins
    b. Anterior jugular vein
    c. Medial cubital vein
    d. Interosseous vein

16. Which of the following forearm vessels are not routinely evaluated during upper extremity venous duplex testing?
    a. Basilic and cephalic veins
    b. Basilic and ulnar veins
    c. Cephalic and radial veins
    d. Radial and ulnar veins

17. A 34-year-old female presents to the vascular lab with a 1-day history of arm swelling and redness. The patient has recently had a PICC line inserted. During the duplex evaluation, the axillary and subclavian veins are incompressible with hypoechoic echoes noted within their lumens. What are these findings consistent with?
    a. Chronic venous thrombosis
    b. Acute venous thrombosis
    c. Acute venous insufficiency
    d. Normal findings in these vessels

18. A 78-year-old male presents to the vascular lab with right arm swelling for the past several days. The patient notes that he is currently being treated for cancer. During the upper extremity duplex exam, decreased pulsatility is noted in the right internal jugular and subclavian veins as well as rouleaux (slow) flow formation. What do these findings suggest?
    a. Normal upper extremity duplex examination
    b. A more distal obstruction, likely in the brachial and cephalic veins
    c. A more proximal obstruction, likely in the brachiocephalic vein or superior vena cava
    d. Congestive heart failure

19. During an upper extremity venous duplex evaluation, color flow is noted filling the axillary vein. However, in a transverse view, the axillary vein is noted to be only partially compressible. Which of the following could explain these findings?
    a. Color priority set too low and color gain too high
    b. Color scale too high and color gain too low
    c. Color priority and scale too high
    d. Color packet size and gain too low

20. A 22-year-old male patient presents to the vascular lab with a 3-day history of left arm swelling with no apparent injury or risk factors. Upon further questioning, the patient does state that he has recently begun weight training. Which of the following should the vascular technologist suspect in this patient?
    a. Effort thrombosis
    b. Superficial venous thrombosis
    c. Superior vena cava syndrome
    d. Lymphedema

FILL-IN-THE-BLANK

1. Signs and symptoms of upper extremity venous thrombosis are similar to those of the leg and can include arm or hand _____, a _____ cord, _____, pain, and _____.

2. The _____ veins of the arm are more affected by venous thrombosis than in the legs.

3. The components of Virchow's Triad include _____, _____, and _____.

4. Thrombosis in the upper extremity veins is now most commonly due to more frequent introduction of _____ and _____ into arm veins.

5. Common veins to use for catheter placement and therefore for venous thrombosis are the _____ vein and the _____ vein. Another common vessel affected by thrombosis due to peripherally inserted central catheter (PICC) placement is the _____ vein.

6. Individuals who present with upper extremity thrombosis secondary to compression of the subclavian vein at the thoracic inlet have what is termed _____ thrombosis or _____ syndrome. These individuals tend to be young, _____, and _____ males.

7. Superior vena cava syndrome often causes facial _____ and dilated _____ collaterals.

8. Asymptomatic patients may present to the vascular lab for upper extremity venous evaluation prior to _____ placement, venous _____ for bypass or other conduit use, and before placement of _____ wires or other cardiac devices.

9. Gentle compression with the transducer is applied over veins in order to cause the walls to _____ or _____ together. Transducer compressions should be repeated every _____ cm along the course of the vein.

10. Compression of the _____ and _____ veins is usually not performed due to the position of these vessels in relation to the _____ and the _____. _____ Doppler and _____ Doppler waveforms should be relied upon to document _____ in those vessels where compression is not possible.

11. To evaluate the internal jugular, brachiocephalic, subclavian, axillary, and brachial veins, a _____ MHz, _____ array transducer is typically used. However, it is helpful to use a _____ MHz transducer when evaluating small forearm veins as well as superficial upper extremity veins.

12. When sitting up or lying with the head elevated, _____ pressure causes the _____ and _____ veins to collapse; therefore, it is preferable to evaluate these vessels with the patient lying _____.

13. Evaluation of the jugular veins should be included in the upper extremity evaluation as they can be involved in the thrombotic process as an _____ from the other upper extremity vessels or as an isolated event due to _____ placement. Additionally, jugular veins can provide _____ pathways in the presence of upper extremity thrombosis.

14. The typical landmark used to identify the internal jugular vein is the _____ artery. Documentation of the internal jugular vein should include _____ images with and without _____, as well as _____ Doppler waveforms.

15. The external jugular vein runs without an _____ and usually terminates into the _____ vein. This vein is also very close to the _____ and is usually found _____ from the view of the internal jugular vein.

16. The confluence of the subclavian and internal jugular veins forms the _____ vein. Evaluation of this vessel should include _____ image demonstrating absence of thrombus, _____ image documenting color filling, and _____ waveforms to show flow characteristics.

17. The _____ vein connects the cephalic and basilic veins. This vein is a common site for thrombus formation because it is a common site for _____.

18. When following the axillary vein through the upper arm, a large, superficial branch will leave it. This vessel is known as the _____ vein. The axillary vein then becomes the _____ vein.

19. The _____, _____, and _____ veins are commonly paired and course with an adjacent artery.

20. Spectral Doppler characteristics of the upper extremity venous system include respiratory _____ and pronounced _____ in the more centrally located vessels.

SHORT ANSWER

1. List the upper extremity vessels that are most routinely evaluated during a venous duplex exam. Which vessels may be added if symptoms or thrombosis are present?

2. Compare and contrast spectral Doppler waveforms from the upper extremity veins and the lower extremity veins.

IMAGE EVALUATION/PATHOLOGY

Review the images and answer the following questions.

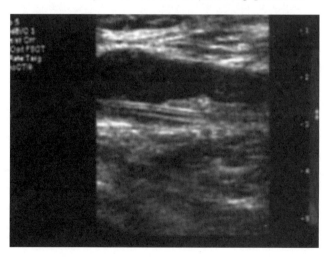

1. A 46-year-old female presented to the vascular lab for evaluation of catheter placement. The above image was obtained during the duplex evaluation. Describe the findings in this image.

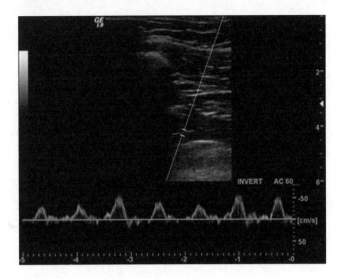

2. Describe the spectral Doppler waveform seen in the above image. Which vessel is this likely taken from?

CASE STUDY

1. A 75-year-old female presents to the vascular lab with right upper extremity swelling for the past 3 to 4 days. She has recently had a PICC line inserted through the cephalic vein. Upon duplex evaluation, the cephalic vein near the PICC line is incompressible and dilated with hypoechoic echoes present in the lumen. Additionally, the distal subclavian vein demonstrates hypoechoic echoes within its lumen and is Doppler silent.

Assuming the brachial and basilic veins are patent, what would the spectral Doppler findings likely be in these vessels?

What other vessels would need to be evaluated in this patient? Given the history and the limited findings above, where else might be suspect for thrombus development? What are some treatment options for this patient?

2. A 19-year-old male presents to the vascular lab for suspected Paget-Schroetter syndrome. What symptoms and history would you expect this patient to have? Which vessel or vessels would be most important to assess in this patient? Why?

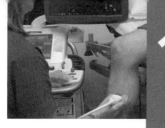

16 Ultrasound Evaluation and Mapping of the Superficial Venous System

REVIEW OF GLOSSARY TERMS

MATCHING

Match the key terms with their definitions.

Key Terms

1. _____ Great saphenous vein
2. _____ Small saphenous vein
3. _____ Perforator vein
4. _____ Mapping
5. _____ Recanalization
6. _____ Varicosities

Definition

a. Dilated, tortuous superficial veins
b. A vein that connects from the superficial venous system to the deep system
c. A superficial vein forming at the level of the medial malleolus; courses along medial calf and thigh
d. A vein that is not patent but had previously been thrombosed
e. A superficial vein that courses along the posterior aspect of the calf, terminating into the popliteal vein
f. Evaluating the patency, position, depth, and size of the superficial venous system for use as bypass conduit or other surgical procedures

ANATOMY AND PHYSIOLOGY REVIEW

IMAGE LABELING

Complete the labels in the images that follow.

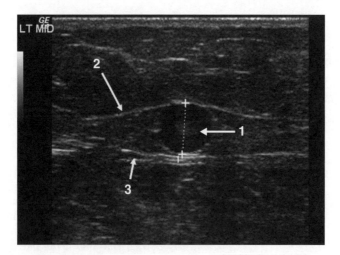

A transverse view through the mid-medial thigh.

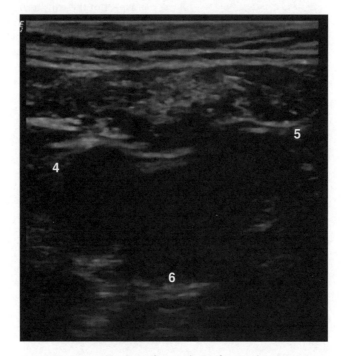

A transverse view at the saphenofemoral junction.

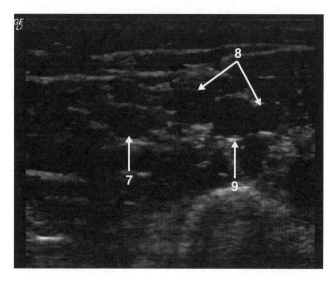

A transverse view through the mid-upper arm.

CHAPTER REVIEW

MULTIPLE CHOICE

Complete each question by circling the best answer.

1. Which of the following characteristics are assessed during preoperative evaluation of the superficial venous system?
   a. Vein patency
   b. Vein depth and size
   c. Vein position
   d. All of the above

2. How many common configurations has the thigh portion of the great saphenous vein been found to have?
   a. 10
   b. 2
   c. 4
   d. 5

3. What is a vein that penetrates the muscular fascia of the leg and connects the superficial system to the deep system?
   a. Accessory saphenous vein
   b. Perforating vein
   c. Deep muscular vein
   d. Venous sinus

4. In order to maximize venous pressure and distention, in what position should the patient's limbs be placed when mapping the superficial venous system?
   a. Dependent
   b. Elevated
   c. Contracted
   d. Adducted

5. Which of the following measures can be taken to ensure a patient's vessels do not vasoconstrict?
   a. Keep the exam room cool and the patient uncovered
   b. Keep the exam room cool but cover the patient, only exposing the limb being evaluated
   c. Keep the exam room warm and cover the patient, only exposing the limb being evaluated
   d. Keep the exam room warm and only cover the foot of the limb being evaluated

6. Since superficial veins are under low pressure and just under the skin, what type of transducer compression must be used to compress these veins?
   a. Light
   b. Heavy
   c. Moderate
   d. Extreme

7. Which of the following describes the proper technique for marking a superficial vein in a longitudinal image orientation?
   a. Vein should appear ovoid in shape; transducer should be perpendicular to skin surface
   b. Vein should appear ovoid in shape; transducer should be oblique to skin surface
   c. Vein should fill screen from left to right; transducer should be perpendicular to skin surface
   d. Vein should fill screen from left to right; transducer should be oblique to skin surface

8. At what distance should marks be placed along the length of the vein when marking?
   a. 2 to 3 in
   b. 2 to 3 cm
   c. 5 to 6 cm
   d. 8 to 9 cm

9. When mapping and marking superficial veins, what is the transverse orientation useful to help identify?
   a. The relationship of superficial veins to deep veins
   b. Branch points and vein diameter
   c. Vein diameter only
   d. Branch points and perforator location only

10. When measuring vein diameters for use as a conduit, where should veins be measured from?
    a. Outer wall to outer wall
    b. Outer wall to inner wall
    c. Inner wall to outer wall
    d. Inner wall to inner wall

11. The superficial veins of the arm are usually easiest to identify in which part of the arm?
    a. Upper arm
    b. Forearm
    c. Near the wrist
    d. At the antecubital fossa

12. In the above question, why are the vessels easier to identify at that level?
    a. The vessels are deeper and smaller in diameter
    b. The vessels are larger and have the least amount of branches
    c. The vessels are more superficial with multiple branches
    d. The vessels follow the deep system

13. Which of the following landmarks can be used to identify the cephalic vein in the upper arm?
    a. Brachial artery
    b. Radial artery
    c. Biceps muscle
    d. Clavicle

14. Which of the following transducer frequencies would be most appropriate for mapping of the cephalic vein?
    a. 7 MHz
    b. 3.5 MHz
    c. 10 MHz
    d. 15 MHz

15. During a vein mapping procedure, the technologist visualizes a portion of the great saphenous vein that is partially compressible with decreased phasicity upon Doppler interrogation. What does this most likely represent?
    a. Acute, occlusive thrombosis
    b. Partial thrombosis of this vein section
    c. Chronic thrombosis of a varicosity
    d. Normal findings in the great saphenous vein

16. Which of the following conditions results in a vein that is unusable as a bypass conduit?
    a. Wall thickening with evidence of recanalization
    b. Vein wall calcifications
    c. Isolated valve abnormalities
    d. All of the above

17. During a venous mapping procedure, the patient notes that she has had prior vein stripping; however, the technologist finds a large superficial vein on the anterior medial aspect of the thigh. What does this most likely represent?
    a. The main great saphenous vein, which has recanalized
    b. The anterior accessory saphenous vein, which has become dominant
    c. The posterior accessory saphenous vein, which has become dominant
    d. A varicosity that should not be evaluated

18. What minimum size should the vein be in order to be used as a conduit?
    a. 1.0 to 2.0 mm
    b. 1.0 to 2.0 cm
    c. 2.5 to 3.0 mm
    d. 1.5 to 2.0 mm

19. During a venous mapping procedure, the technologist notes a thin, echogenic line protruding into the vessel lumen that does not appear to be mobile. The patient does not have a history of previous superficial thrombophlebitis. What does this finding likely represent?
    a. Chronic thrombosis
    b. Stenotic, frozen valve
    c. Vein wall calcification
    d. Varicosity

20. When using color and spectral Doppler to evaluate the superficial venous system, which of the following settings should be used?
    a. High gain and high PRF/scale
    b. Low gain and high PRF/scale
    c. Low gain and low PRF/scale
    d. High gain and low PRF/scale

FILL-IN-THE-BLANK

1. The most common uses for superficial veins as conduits are for _____ bypass grafting, _____ bypass grafting, and _____ fistula.

2. The limitations of superficial venous mapping include patient _____, _____, and _____.

3. Mapping is used to determine the suitability of the vein as a conduit in terms of vein _____, _____, _____, and _____.

4. The _____ _____ vein is the standard name for the vein, which had been referred to as the greater or long saphenous vein. The _____ _____ vein is the standard name for the vein previously known as the lesser or short saphenous vein.

5. When using a superficial vein for in situ arterial bypass, _____ veins must always be identified and ligated. If these vessels are not ligated, a _____ can be formed.

6. The cephalic vein courses up the _____ side of the forearm; the basilic vein courses up the _____ side of the forearm; these two vessels communicate at the antecubital fossa via the _____ _____ vein.

7. The main great saphenous vein is typically bounded superficially by the _____ _____ and deeply by the _____ _____. This creates an _____ eye appearance when viewed in transverse.

8. There are several common configurations on the great saphenous vein. The majority of the time, there is a _____ trunk, which runs _____ in the thigh.

9. When a double saphenous system occurs, it is important to distinguish which system is _____ so the surgeon can select appropriately. Often, the two systems have many _____ that also must be noted.

10. The _____ _____ vein is typically a _____ trunk that courses up the middle of the posterior aspect of the calf and terminates into the _____ vein.

11. When mapping directly onto the patient's skin, the patient should avoid body _____ and the technologist should limit the use of _____ and cover the transducer with a _____.

12. The optimal patient position for mapping of the great saphenous vein is a _____ _____ position with the hip _____ rotated and knee _____.

13. When starting to map the great saphenous vein, it can be identified at the _____ junction in a _____ orientation using _____ probe pressure.

14. If using a longitudinal approach to vein mapping, the technologist should be sure that the vein _____ the screen from right to left and that the transducer is _____ to the skin surface. If using the transverse plane, the vein should appear _____ and _____ on the ultrasound screen.

15. When mapping a vein, vein _____ should be measured and two types of branches should be identified: _____ branches and deep _____ veins.

16. When measuring vein diameter, calipers should be placed along the _____ vein wall and the _____. This results in a(n) _____ vein size when compared to intraoperative measurements.

17. Appropriate system settings for venous mapping include adjusting the transmit power and focal zones for a well-defined _____ field image; use of a transducer frequency of at least _____ MHz; and adjusting Doppler settings to detect _____.

18. A normal, healthy vein should have _____, _____ walls and be easily _____ with minimal transducer pressure. Additionally, valve sinuses should be _____ in shape with freely moving valve _____.

19. Acute thrombus is usually _____ or _____ in echogenicity, whereas chronic thrombus may be _____. Superficial veins that are thrombosed demonstrate lack of _____ with transducer pressure On Doppler, thrombosed veins demonstrate a lack of _____ filling with no _____ signal/waveform.

20. Veins presenting with an _____ intimal surface or wall _____ may indicate evidence of _____. These veins are/are not considered adequate for conduit for bypass.

SHORT ANSWER

1. Describe the characteristics of a normal, healthy vein that may be used for mapping. What vein diameter is optimal and why?

2. Describe the common configurations of the great saphenous vein, small saphenous vein, cephalic vein, and basilic vein.

3. List the standardized nomenclature for the superficial venous system of the lower extremity. Include the historic name as a reference.

IMAGE EVALUATION/PATHOLOGY

Review the images and answer the following questions.

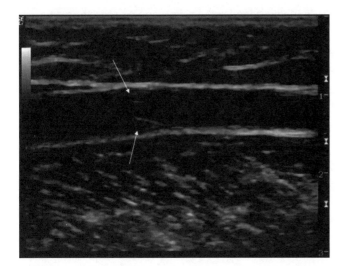

1. The above image demonstrates the saphenofemoral junction. Describe the findings indicated by the white arrows.

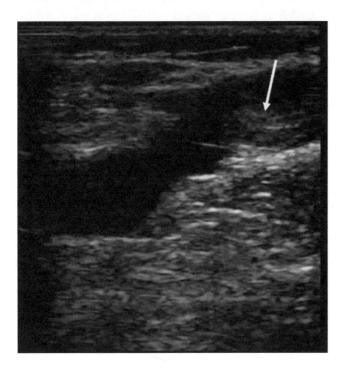

2. Describe the findings demonstrated in the image to the left. Would this vein be adequate for use as a conduit for arterial bypass?

CASE STUDY

Review the information and answer the following questions.

1. A 66-year-old male presents to the vascular lab for lower extremity vein mapping prior to right femoral–popliteal arterial bypass grafting. During the procedure, the right great saphenous vein demonstrates evidence of segmental chronic venous thrombosis. What options may the surgeon have in this case? What additional vessels would be appropriate to evaluate?

2. You have completed a vein mapping procedure on a 75-year-old female and have the following findings: left great saphenous vein measures 2.8 to 3.3 mm in the thigh and 1.6 to 2.5 mm in the calf; right great saphenous vein measures 1.9 to 2.4 mm in the thigh and 1.3 to 1.9 mm in the calf; left small saphenous measures 0.9 to 1.2 mm; and right small saphenous measures 1.7 to 2.1 mm. Which vein segments would you recommend for use to your vascular surgeon for lower extremity bypass grafting? What techniques could be used to help ensure maximum dilation of the veins?

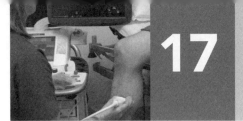

REVIEW OF GLOSSARY TERMS

MATCHING

Match the key terms with their definitions.

Key Terms

1. _____ Reticular veins

2. _____ Varicose veins

3. _____ Telangiectasia

4. _____ CEAP

5. _____ Chronic venous insufficiency

6. _____ Reflux

7. _____ Lymphedema

8. _____ Lipedema

9. _____ Spider vein

10. _____ Vein of Giacomini

Definition

a. Swelling attributed to fat tissue

b. Clinical, etiologic, anatomic, and pathophysiologic classification of chronic venous insufficiency

c. Inadequate name for purple or red telangiectasias, an arteriovenous rather than a venous disorder

d. Veins with a diameter smaller than 3 mm

e. Swelling attributed to lymph channels or lymph node disorders

f. Veins with diameter equal to or greater than 3 mm

g. Long-lasting venous valvular or obstructive disorder

h. Reverse flow, usually in veins with incompetent valves

i. Communicating vein between the great and small saphenous veins

j. Dilation of red, blue, or purple superficial capillaries, arterioles, or venules

CHAPTER REVIEW

MULTIPLE CHOICE

Complete each question by circling the best answer.

1. In which population are varicose veins typically more common?
   a. Men
   b. Women
   c. Varicose veins occur as frequently in men as women
   d. Men over age 65

2. What are other causes of leg edema that may mimic venous obstruction or valvular insufficiency?
   a. Lymphatic obstruction
   b. Cardiac disorders
   c. Lipedema
   d. All of the above

3. A patient presents to the vascular lab with visible spider veins. Based on this information, what would this patient's clinical CEAP classification likely be?
   a. C0
   b. C1
   c. C2
   d. C3

4. A patient presents to the vascular lab with chronic bilateral leg swelling. Upon duplex assessment of the venous system, the deep system was found to be unremarkable, although there was reflux demonstrated in the bilateral great saphenous veins. What is the most likely CEAP classification for this patient?
   a. C3EpAsPr
   b. C2EsApPo
   c. C3EcAsPro
   d. C6EpAsPro

5. Venous pressure in the legs in a supine individual is _____ mm Hg at its highest while it increases to about _____ mm Hg with standing, depending on a person's height.
   a. 25, 200
   b. 10, 20
   c. 10, 100
   d. 50, 120

6. In the above question, what is the reason for the increase in venous pressure with standing?
   a. Cardiac pulsatility
   b. The affect of valves on venous flow
   c. Systolic pressure gradients
   d. Introduction of hydrostatic pressure

7. A true saphenous vein can be determined due to its position within which of the following?
   a. Deep muscular fascia
   b. Subdural lipid layer
   c. Saphenous fascia
   d. Anterior vascular compartment

8. Which of the following is aligned with the deep system?
   a. Anterior accessory saphenous vein
   b. Great saphenous vein
   c. Posterior accessory saphenous vein
   d. Small saphenous vein

9. Into which of the following vessels does the small saphenous vein terminate?
   a. Popliteal vein
   b. Gastrocnemius vein
   c. Distal femoral vein
   d. Any of the above

10. Before assessing the venous system for insufficiency/reflux, which of the following should be performed?
    a. Evaluation of the deep venous system for obstruction or thrombosis
    b. Evaluation of the arterial system for atherosclerotic development
    c. Mapping of the superficial venous system
    d. Auscultation for bruits in the lower extremities

11. In order to best demonstrate valvular incompetence, which position should the patient be examined in?
    a. Supine
    b. Reverse Trendelenburg
    c. Standing
    d. Trendelenburg

12. When performing an exam for CVVI, patency and flow characteristics should be documented at all of the following locations EXCEPT:
    a. Common femoral vein
    b. Femoral vein
    c. Popliteal vein
    d. Anterior tibial vein

13. Which of the following techniques should be used to quantify reflux flow patterns?
    a. B-mode imaging with B flow
    b. Color flow Doppler
    c. Spectral Doppler
    d. Power Doppler

14. Pathologic flow or reflux occurs during _____ of an automatic cuff when the cuff is distal to the site of insonation.
    a. Compression
    b. Decompression
    c. Application
    d. None of the above

15. Which of the following describes the proper use of an automatic cuff compression device?
    a. Rapid inflation from 70 to 80 mm Hg of pressure, held for a few seconds and released quickly
    b. Paced inflation from 70 to 80 mm Hg of pressure, then released quickly
    c. Rapid inflation from 120 mm Hg with immediate rapid deflation
    d. Gradual inflation and deflation of the cuff with the patient's respiratory cycle

16. What is the major advantage of using hand compression instead of automatic cuff inflators?
    a. Reproducibility
    b. Adaptability to unusual venous segments
    c. Standardized technique and pressures
    d. Less technical error

17. Which of the following is NOT a pitfall in measuring reflux?
    a. High persistence resulting in false-positive color flow findings
    b. High-velocity scale or PRF setting affecting color flow sensitivity
    c. Low-wall filter settings allowing visualization of low-velocity venous flow
    d. Gain settings too high altering the sensitivity of spectral Doppler

18. After thermal ablation of a vein, the sonographic findings may include which of the following?
    a. Smooth, thin-walled veins that are fully compressible with anechoic lumens
    b. Dilated, incompressible veins with hypoechoic material filling the vein
    c. Small-diameter vein that is partially compressible with an echogenic lumen
    d. Potentially sonographically absent, fibrosed, or recanalized veins at different locations along the vein length

19. Valvular reflux times as measured on a spectral Doppler display are typically considered abnormal when greater than how many seconds?
    a. 1
    b. 2
    c. 3
    d. 4

20. What is the main purpose for venous photoplethysmography of the lower limb?
    a. Definitive diagnosis of venous reflux
    b. Determination of level of reflux
    c. Screening for detection of reflux
    d. Screening for venous thrombosis

21. What can the use of a tourniquet during venous PPG testing help determine?
    a. Deep versus superficial venous reflux
    b. Great saphenous versus accessory saphenous vein reflux
    c. Venous reflux versus venous thrombosis
    d. Perforating vein reflux

22. A patient presents to the vascular laboratory for evaluation of valvular incompetence. A venous PPG examination is performed. The results of the examination demonstrate a venous refill time (VRT) of 10.5 seconds without the use of a tourniquet and 22 seconds with the use of a tourniquet. What do these findings demonstrate?
    a. Normal findings
    b. Presence of deep venous reflux
    c. Presence of superficial venous reflux
    d. Presence of both deep and superficial venous reflux

23. What is air plethysmography useful for?
    a. Determining deep versus superficial venous thrombosis
    b. Determining deep versus superficial venous reflux
    c. Qualification of deep venous reflux
    d. Quantification of chronic venous insufficiency

24. Using APG, increased ambulatory pressures suggestive of the inability to empty the calf veins due to poor or nonfunctional calf muscle pump are indicated with the which of the following findings?
    a. Residual volume greater than 20% to 35%
    b. Low venous volume
    c. Venous filling rate less than 2 ml/sec
    d. Venous filling time greater than 25 seconds

25. Which of the following is an emerging technology that may help with guidance of venous access, phlebotomy, and injection sclerotherapy?
    a. Venous photophlethysmography
    b. Near-infrared imaging
    c. Air plethysmography
    d. Radiofrequency imaging

FILL-IN-THE-BLANK

1. Chronic venous insufficiency (CVI) is a term used to describe venous insufficiency due to venous _____ or _____ insufficiency, whereas chronic venous valvular insufficiency (CVVI), a subset of CVI, deals only with _____.

2. Along with the great and small saphenous veins, the vascular technologist must also be familiar with the _____ and _____ accessory saphenous veins and the vein of _____.

3. Saphenous veins are within a saphenous _____, readily identifying them on ultrasound. This structure gives the saphenous veins their distinctive _____ appearance.

4. The landmark to identify the anterior accessory saphenous vein is the _____, which is a vertical line perpendicular to the transducer surface that runs through the _____ artery and vein.

5. _____ are veins that drain into another major vein. These vessels pierce the saphenous _____ and drain into the corresponding saphenous vein.

6. An ultrasound landmark used to identify the GSV below the knee is the "_____ _____." This is a triangle

formed by the _____ muscle, the _____ bone, and the _____ _____ vein.

7. The GSV and common femoral vein confluence is termed the _____ _____. Several tributaries join the GSV at this level, including the superficial _____ vein, the _____ external _____ vein, and the _____ _____ iliac vein.

8. The confluence of the short saphenous vein and the deep venous system is variable. It may terminate into the _____ vein at the _____ junction, the _____ vein, the distal _____ vein of the thigh, or various other unnamed and/or perforating veins.

9. Venous valves are _____ leaflet valves that point _____ of normal venous drainage. Incompetent valves permit _____ flow or reflux.

10. The highest rate of prevalence of reflux is found in the _____ _____ vein. Prevalence tends to increase with severity of _____ _____ and with increasing _____.

11. Visual signs of abnormal venous pressures that are the primary basis for CEAP classification include _____ veins, _____, _____ veins, _____ veins, _____, _____ changes, and _____.

12. Phleboedema is often described by the patient as temporary leg _____ at the end of a working day, after prolonged _____, or as a consequence of certain _____ or leg _____.

13. Differential diagnosis of edema includes _____ obstruction, _____ disease, _____ disease, sympathetic _____, or _____ disorders.

14. Skin changes that are often associated with CVVI include localized _____, atrophic _____, corona _____, _____ (hardening of the skin), and _____ (healed or not).

15. Symptoms commonly described by patients with CVVI include _____, tension, aching, _____, _____ legs, muscle _____, _____, discomfort, _____, _____, itching, and skin _____ or _____.

16. A patient with open skin ulcers, CVVI as major cause of clinical manifestations, and affecting superficial and perforating veins with a pathological combination of pathophysiology would have a CEAP classification of _____.

17. Additional classification systems that may be used to quantify and describe CVVI symptoms and severity include the Clinical _____ Score, the _____ Score and the _____ of _____ Questionnaires.

18. Duplex Doppler ultrasonography has two major diagnostic goals for CVVI: first is to rule out _____ _____ _____ and the second is the evaluation of _____ _____ (reflux detection).

19. Treatment options for CVVI include _____, _____ (associated with "neovascularization"), thermal _____, _____ (chemical ablation), and _____ (microincision).

20. Endovenous _____ _____ by radio _____ or _____ energy has largely replaced stripping and ligation as the treatment of choice for CVVI. This procedure causes _____ injury to the treated vein segments. Over time, the treated segments will gradually _____ and then _____.

21. Patient positioning for evaluation for venous disease typically starts with the patient in _____ _____ position for evaluation of deep veins, whereas a _____ position is recommended for evaluation of CVVI. This second position allows for optimal _____ and venous _____.

22. Prior to evaluating the venous system for evidence of valvular insufficiency, evaluation for _____ or _____ venous obstruction should be performed. If _____ venous thrombosis is found, evaluation for CVVI is _____. If _____ venous obstruction is found, CVVI evaluation is _____.

23. After the venous systems are found to be patent, determination of _____ _____ using spectral Doppler is performed. Compression techniques are used to assess reflux. When using proper compression techniques, normal veins proximal to the site of compression should demonstrate _____ flow during compression with _____ during decompression; however, abnormal veins proximal to the site of compression would demonstrate _____ flow during compression with _____ flow during decompression.

24. Compression maneuvers can be accomplished by several methods. The most reproducible include _____ cuff _____/_____ and the "_____ _____." A less reproducible method that offers more flexibility is _____ compression. The _____ maneuver is also commonly used for large, proximal veins.

25. Reflux time measurement should be performed with _____ Doppler with the vein in a _____ image. _____ Doppler in a _____ image can be used for screening or detection of severe reflux but should be validated with _____ Doppler.

26. When performing a screening exam for CVVI, the protocol should include documentation of the _____ (deep) veins and single documentation of _____ (superficial) vein abnormalities. This type of scan focuses primarily on the region of _____ _____ of an abnormality.

27. For definitive diagnosis of CVVI, at least three variations of protocol exist. First, there is a protocol for selection of patients for _____ _____ of the GSV in the thigh. Second, patients could be examined in a phlebology clinic with _____ ultrasound capabilities. This protocol is performed at the time of _____. Last is the examination of patients for limited or extensive _____/_____ /_____ procedures.

28. When performing the third type of protocol for definitive diagnosis, extensive documentation is performed, including drawing of _____ and non_____ veins plus documentation of _____ veins and _____ and _____ points of reflux.

29. The use of ultrasound during treatment for CVVI includes use during thermal _____ to map the course of the vein and to visualize _____, introducers, _____, and laser or radiofrequency _____. Ultrasound can also be used during foam _____ to visualize needle _____ and foam as it travels through the vein.

30. During postablation follow-up, the most important ultrasound documentation should be of the _____ veins to assure patency. Follow-up is also used to examine the _____ vein to demonstrate if veins are fully _____ or if there is _____.

31. To detect reflux, system settings should be adjusted to detect _____ flow. This may include _____ gain, _____ persistence, and _____ velocity scales (PRF).

32. Diagnostic criteria for CVVI include B-mode characteristics of _____ of vein diameter and valve sinuses with _____ valve leaflets plus PW spectral and color flow Doppler documentation of _____ flow following _____ compression or release of _____ compression.

33. Venous photoplethysmography is mainly used as a _____ procedure for the detection of reflux. A PPG transducer is placed on the _____ aspect of the calf and _____ refill _____ is measured after the patient performs 5 to 10 foot _____ maneuvers. Normal recovery time is greater than _____ seconds.

34. Air plethysmography is a recommended technique for _____ of chronic venous insufficiency. APG can be used to differentiate _____ cause of CVVI from aesthetic problems, demonstrate and quantify disease _____, and to show quantifiable _____ pre- and posttreatment.

35. The parameters measured by APG include venous _____ , filling _____, venous _____ rate, and _____ volume. Low VV may indicate venous _____ , whereas a high VV may indicate venous _____. An FT that is shorter than 25 seconds indicates _____ . An FR greater than 2 ml/sec indicates venous _____, whereas an RV percentage greater than 20% to 35% suggests increased ambulatory venous _____.

SHORT ANSWER

1. What are the differences in protocol for a screening exam for valvular insufficiency and an exam designed for definitive diagnosis?

2. List and briefly describe the treatment types available for CVVI.

3. What is the role of photo and air plethysmography in the diagnosis of CVVI?

IMAGE EVALUATION/PATHOLOGY

Review the images and answer the following questions.

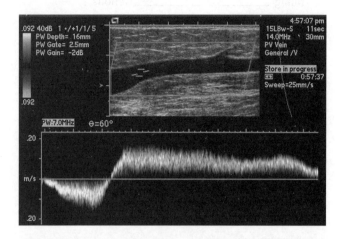

1. This image was taken in the great saphenous vein just distal to the saphenofemoral junction. The patient was asked to perform a Valsalva maneuver and this image was the result. Explain the findings and if they are significant.

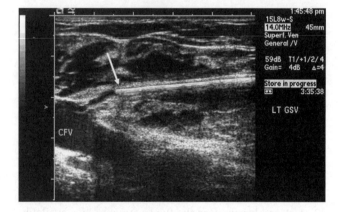

2. This image is of the left great saphenous vein just distal to the saphenofemoral junction. Describe the structure the white arrow is pointing to. What is its purpose?

CASE STUDY

Review the information and answer the following questions.

1. 44-year-old female presents to the vascular lab with the following CEAP classification: C2EpAsPr. She has been referred for verification of this classification by duplex testing. Explain the CEAP classification for this patient. What duplex protocol would be most appropriate for this patient, and what would you expect the findings to be?

2. A 52-year-old female presented to the vascular lab for varicose vein evaluation. Findings during the evaluation were as follows:

   Right GSV: visually enlarged and tortuous with retrograde flow lasting 750 ms, retrograde flow also visualized with color throughout entire length

Left GSV: visually appears to have normal diameter; minimal retrograde flow (< 350 ms)

Right femoropopliteal segments: thickened vessel walls with mostly anechoic lumens that are not fully compressible with transducer compression and retrograde flow noted at 1.2 sec

Left femoropopliteal segments: anechoic lumens that are compressible with transducer compression with minimal retrograde flow (<0.5 sec)

Which vessel(s) demonstrate reflux? Of the vessels that demonstrate reflux, what is likely the underlying pathophysiology?

3. A 67-year-old male presents to the vascular lab for venous APG testing. A standard APG test is performed with the following results:

Venous volume = 200 mL

Venous filling time = 10 seconds

Venous filling rate = 2.5 mL/sec

Residual volume percentage = 37%

What do these results suggest? What further testing, if any, should be suggested in this patient?

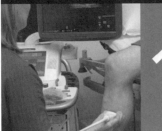

18 Aorta and Iliac Arteries

REVIEW OF GLOSSARY TERMS

MATCHING

Match the key terms with their definitions.

Key Terms

1. _____ Aneurysm

2. _____ Fusiform

3. _____ Saccular

4. _____ Endoleak

5. _____ EVAR

Definitions

a. Asymmetric outpouching dilations of a vessel, often caused by trauma or penetrating aortic ulcers

b. Persistent blood flow demonstrated outside of a stent graft endovascular repair but within aneurysm sac

c. A focal dilation of an artery involving all three layers of the vessel wall that exceeds the normal diameter by more than 50%

d. Placement of a stent graft within an aortic aneurysm sac via a catheter as a means of repair

e. Circumferential dilation of a vessel involving all three vessel walls

ANATOMY AND PHYSIOLOGY REVIEW

IMAGE LABELING

Complete the labels in the images that follow.

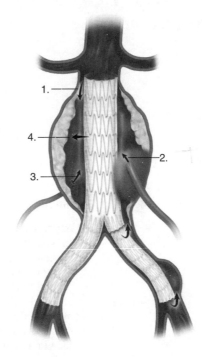

The types of endoleaks in the above image.

CHAPTER REVIEW

MULTIPLE CHOICE

Complete each question by circling the best answer.

1. Popliteal aneurysms are associated with abdominal aortic aneurysms at about what rate?
   a. 10%
   b. 20%
   c. 30%
   d. 50%

2. In which of the following patients would an abdominal aortic aneurysm most likely be found?
   a. A 69-year-old male
   b. A 75-year-old female
   c. A 37-year-old male
   d. A 28-year-old female

3. What is the indication to evaluate the aortoiliac segments known as blue toe syndrome caused by?
   a. Vasospasm
   b. Small vessel occlusive disease
   c. Cold sensitivity
   d. Embolic events

4. Which of the following patient preparation steps should be taken in order to reduce overlying bowel gas before an aortoiliac duplex evaluation?
   a. Take medication for gas reduction
   b. Fast overnight
   c. No specific preparation is necessary
   d. Chew gum

5. What position can the sonographer assume in order to help relieve strain on the arm and/or elbow when applying pressure to view the aorta and iliac arteries?
   a. Position shoulder over the transducer to allow body weight to help push
   b. Abduct arm to reach across the patient
   c. Bend at waist and extend arm to better visualize iliac vessels
   d. Position flexed wrist over transducer and push from the shoulder

6. In order to visualize the deep vessels of the abdomen, what frequency transducer is most commonly used?
   a. 7 to 10 MHz
   b. 2 to 5 MHz
   c. 5 to 8 MHz
   d. 1 to 2 MHz

7. What is the most common location for abdominal aortic aneurysms?
   a. Suprarenal
   b. At the level of the superior mesenteric artery
   c. Infrarenal
   d. Proximal aorta just as it passes through the diaphragm

8. Which of the following is NOT associated with normal findings in the abdominal aorta?
   a. Smooth margins
   b. Tapering distally
   c. Tortuosity near the bifurcation
   d. No focal dilatation

9. The abdominal aorta is considered aneurysmal when the diameter measures greater than what?
   a. 1 cm
   b. 2 cm
   c. 3 cm
   d. 3 mm

10. What shape are most aortic aneurysms?
    a. Fusiform
    b. Saccular
    c. Mycotic
    d. Dissecting

11. As an abdominal aortic aneurysm enlarges, what does it also have a tendency to do?
    a. Elongate
    b. Foreshorten
    c. Straighten
    d. Constrict

12. In order to get the most accurate diameter measurement of the abdominal aorta, the technologist should be sure to align the transducer in what relation to the vessel?
    a. Parallel
    b. Oblique
    c. Perpendicular
    d. Sagittally

13. When viewing the abdominal aorta in transverse, which dimension provides the most accurate diameter measurement?
    a. Anterior to posterior
    b. Right to left lateral
    c. Superior to inferior
    d. All are equally accurate

14. During an aortoiliac duplex examination, the distal aorta measures 2.5 cm in diameter. What are these findings consistent with?
    a. Normal aortic dimension
    b. Aortic ectasia
    c. Aortic aneurysm
    d. Aortic dissection

15. When an abdominal aortic aneurysm is found, which of the following additional parameters should be included?
    a. Length of aneurysm
    b. Proximity of aneurysm to renal arteries
    c. Presence and extent of any intraluminal thrombus
    d. All of the above

16. What landmark is used to determine the end of the common iliac artery and beginning of the external iliac artery?
    a. Inguinal ligament
    b. Origin of internal iliac artery
    c. Umbilicus
    d. Iliac crest

17. What is an important reason to follow up with patients after aortoiliac intervention with duplex ultrasound?
    a. Follow-up and treatment of restenosis may improve patency rates
    b. Occlusion is easier to manage than stenoses
    c. Angioplasty and stenting do not have significant restenosis rates
    d. Duplex ultrasound is not used for follow-up

18. When evaluating a stent within the aortoiliac system, which of the following is FALSE?
    a. Stent alignment should be visualized
    b. Full deployment of stent should be documented
    c. Relationship of stent to vessel wall is needed
    d. Evaluation of the vessel distal to the stent is not needed

19. A 65-year-old male presents to the vascular lab for evaluation of the abdomen after involvement in a car accident. During the duplex exam, an asymmetric outpouching is identified in the mid to distal aorta. What are these findings consistent with?
    a. Fusiform aneurysm
    b. Saccular aneurysm
    c. Aortic dissection
    d. Aortic stenosis

20. Upon duplex evaluation of a known abdominal aortic aneurysm, homogeneous echoes with smooth borders are visualized with the aneurysm sac. What are these findings consistent with?
    a. Calcifications
    b. Atherosclerotic plaque
    c. Thrombus formation
    d. Vessel dissection

21. A 72-year-old male presents to the vascular lab for follow-up after common iliac stenting. Upon examination, the stent in the mid common iliac artery is elliptical in shape. What does this appearance likely indicate?
    a. Partial stent compression
    b. Normally deployed stent
    c. A kink within the stent
    d. Vessel dissection in the area of the stent

22. During Doppler evaluation of the abdominal aorta, two flow channels are noted. What is this finding consistent with?
    a. Fusiform aneurysm
    b. Saccular aneurysm
    c. Aortic dissection
    d. Aortic stenosis

23. A 76-year-old female patient presents to the vascular lab with left hip and buttock claudication. During the duplex evaluation, velocities in the distal common iliac artery are 72 cm/sec, while velocities in the proximal external iliac artery are 302 cm/s. Which of the following are these findings are likely consistent with?
    a. >50% stenosis in the proximal external iliac artery
    b. <50% stenosis in the proximal external iliac artery
    c. >50% in the distal common iliac artery
    d. External iliac artery dissection

24. Which of the following is NOT a benefit of endovascular stent graft repair of AAA?
    a. Lower perioperative mortality
    b. Decreased survival rates over open surgical repair
    c. Shorter recovery time
    d. Lack of abdominal incision

25. What is the goal of EVAR?
    a. Reduce the size of the aortic lumen
    b. Occlude the aorta in order to avoid aortic rupture
    c. Exclude the aneurysm sac from the general circulation
    d. Increase the size of the aorta to treat stenosis

26. Which of the following can color Doppler ultrasound monitoring of EVAR demonstrate?
    a. Residual sac size
    b. Graft limb dysfunction and kinking
    c. Hemodynamics within the graft site
    d. All of the above

27. Which of the following is the most frequently deployed stent graft device?
    a. Bifurcated
    b. Straight tube
    c. Uni-iliac graft
    d. Fenestrated grafts

28. During the evaluation of an aortic stent graft, the vascular technologist notes a hyperechoic signal along the anterior and posterior walls of the aortic lumen just below the level of the renal arteries. What is this finding consistent with?
    a. Kinking of the stent graft
    b. Normal findings of the proximal attachment site
    c. Endoleak at the proximal graft site
    d. Graft bifurcation at the distal attachment site

29. Which of the following is NOT an indication of aneurysm sac instability after EVAR?
    a. Increase in sac size
    b. Pulsatility of the sac
    c. Decrease in size of aneurysm sac
    d. Areas of echolucency within the sac

30. An 80-year-old male presents for follow-up after endovascular treatment of his AAA. During the evaluation, the stent graft is identified and appears to be in a correct position by B-mode; however, the aortic diameter is 5.5 cm compared to 4.9 cm on previous examination. Doppler evaluation is then performed, and flow is identified along the posterior aorta outside the stent graft material. What are these findings consistent with?
    a. Kinking of the stent graft material
    b. Stent graft endoleak
    c. Migration of the stent graft causing stenosis
    d. Normal findings after stent graft placement

FILL-IN-THE-BLANK

1. Limitations that may prevent the complete evaluation of the aortoiliac arterial segments during ultrasound evaluation include recent ____________ surgery, open ____________, indwelling ____________, or ____________.

2. Iliac arteries are considered aneurysmal when the diameter increases more than ____________% compared to an ____________ segment or generally when the diameter exceeds ____________ cm. Iliac artery aneurysms are usually associated with ____________ disease and are often ____________.

3. Complications of iliac aneurysms can include ____________, ____________, or ____________ compression.

4. In preparation for aortoiliac duplex, the patient should fast ____________ to minimize the effects of ____________ gas. During the procedure, the patient should be ____________ in a comfortable position with the head ____________.

5. Indications for aortoiliac duplex ultrasound include ____________ abdominal ____________, suspected or known aortic or iliac ____________ disease, ____________ (usually of hip or buttock area), decreased femoral ____________, abdominal ____________, and ____________ toe ____________.

6. Ultrasound evaluation of the aorta and iliac vessels should begin at the level of the ____________ and extend to the ____________ bifurcation, with evaluation in both the ____________ and ____________ planes.

7. The normal aorta lies immediately adjacent to the ____________, has ____________ margins, no focal ____________, and ____________ toward the level of the ____________.

8. When performing diameter measurements of the aorta, care must be taken to ensure that the transducer is ____________ or ____________ to the aorta itself, especially in the event of aortic neck ____________.

9. In addition to documenting aortic diameter measurements in the presence of focal dilatation, it is also important to note dilatation ____________, proximity to the ____________ arteries, and the presence and ____________ of any intraluminal ____________.

10. All spectral Doppler waveforms are collected maintaining an angle of ____________ degrees or less ____________ to the vessel wall and with the sample ____________ placed in the ____________ stream of the vessel.

11. Careful duplex assessment of the aortoiliac vessels can determine if disease is ____________ or ____________; the ____________, length, and ____________ of lesions; and help determine residual ____________.

12. When performing a comprehensive, preintervention aortoiliac duplex exam, the study should include evaluation of the entire ____________,

_____ vessel origins,

_____, _____,

and _____ iliac arteries as

well as common, superficial, and profunda

_____ arteries.

13. Following intervention, duplex follow-up

    becomes important because identification

    and treatment of _____

    prior to complete _____

    may improve _____ rates,

    _____ are technically easier to

    manage, and percutaneous _____

    and _____ procedures are

    associated with significant _____

    rates.

14. During duplex evaluation of stent

    placement, it is important to evaluate

    for stent _____, full

    stent _____, and

    _____ to the vessel wall. It is also

    important to know stent placement in order to walk

    the _____ throughout the entire

    _____ of the stent.

15. Because the iliac vessels are typically deep and

    _____, _____

    Doppler is often useful to visualize these vessels to

    help obtain proper _____ Doppler

    alignment.

16. An abdominal aneurysm is defined as a

    focal _____ of the aortic

    wall by more than _____

    % or _____ cm.

    _____ is present when

    areas of _____ are less than

    _____ cm or when the aorta

    demonstrates _____ margins and

    a non_____ profile.

17. Most aortic aneurysms are _____,

    which involve the entire _____

    of the vessel wall. Fewer aneurysms are

    _____ in nature, described as

    an _____ outpouching dilation

    and are often caused by _____

    or _____ aortic

    _____.

18. _____ occur when a tear

    forms between _____

    of the vessel wall, usually the

    _____-_____

    interface. _____ dissections

    are identified by _____

    channels of _____, whereas

    _____ dissections may be more

    difficult to visualize due to _____

    in the _____ lumen.

19. When evaluating the hemodynamics in

    the aorta, the proximal aorta demonstrates

    _____-resistance

    characteristics, whereas the distal aorta

    demonstrates _____-resistance

    characteristics. The iliac vessels demonstrate

    _____ flow with

    _____ of flow in early diastole.

20. Defining characteristics of a greater than

    _____% stenosis include

    a velocity ratio of _____:

    _____ when comparing the peak

    _____ velocity in the stenosis

    to the velocity in a _____

    segment. Additionally, post_____

    _____ must be present in order to

    prove a stenosis exists.

21. Chronic _____ in the iliac arterial system can be difficult to visualize because the artery can become _____ and _____. A helpful technique is to follow the companion _____.

22. Endovascular stent _____ repair of AAA is a less _____ procedure with lower perioperative _____ and improved _____ rates, as well as a shorter _____ time when compared to the traditional method.

23. Color duplex ultrasound is often now used as a first choice method of _____ post-EVAR. Ultrasound has the ability to identify _____ and determine leak _____, detect graft limb _____ and _____, and _____ of the stent graft device.

24. When evaluating a stent graft with ultrasound, documentation should include _____ and _____ extent of the graft, _____ measurements of the residual aneurysm _____, B-mode characterization of any _____ or other areas of hypo- or hyper_____, and spectral and color _____ of the aorta, the entire graft, and distal attachment looking for _____ flow, graft _____, thrombosis, or _____.

25. A key to identifying endoleak is a spectral Doppler flow pattern that is _____ from the aortic endograft. When documenting endoleak, it is important to identify the _____ of the leak and the flow _____. Signs of endoleak include increasing _____ size, _____ of the sac, or areas of _____ within the sac on B-mode.

SHORT ANSWER

1. Compare and contrast the protocols for AAA evaluation, preintervention aortoiliac evaluation, and postintervention aortoiliac evaluation.

2. What are the common technical considerations and pitfalls associated with evaluation of the aorta and iliac vessels?

3. Why is close surveillance necessary after EVAR, and what is color duplex ultrasound imaging's role in this process?

IMAGE EVALUATION/PATHOLOGY

Review the images and answer the following questions.

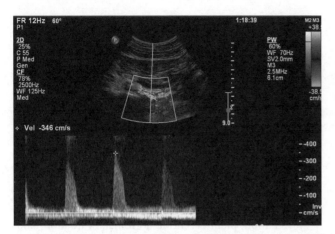 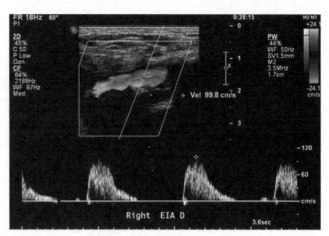

1. The above images were taken from the right external iliac artery. What are your findings?

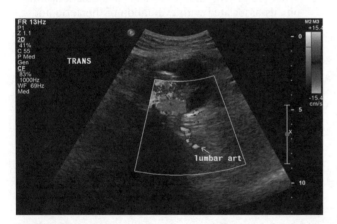 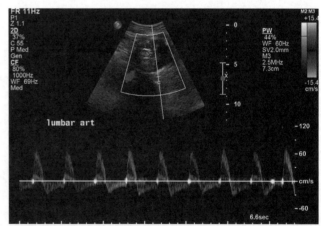

2. The above images were taken on follow-up of EVAR. Describe the findings from these images.

CASE STUDY

Review the information and answer the following questions.

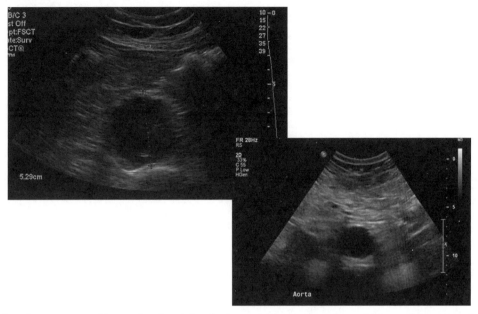

1. A 64-year-old male presents with a pulsatile abdominal mass. The patient has a history of hypertension and smoking. The images were taken during his duplex ultrasound evaluation. What is demonstrated in this patient? Are the ultrasound findings consistent with the patient's clinical presentation?

2. A 67-year-old male presents to the vascular lab for follow-up following recent endovascular stent graft repair of his AAA. Upon questioning, the patient states that he has noticed pain and a pulsatile mass in his left groin. What is the likely cause of the pain and pulsatility in this patient's groin? What documentation should be recorded during this patient's duplex ultrasound evaluation?

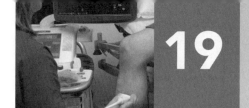

19 The Mesenteric Arteries

REVIEW OF GLOSSARY TERMS

MATCHING

Match the key terms with their definitions.

Key Terms

1. _____ Splanchnic

2. _____ Visceral

3. _____ Postprandial

4. _____ Mesenteric ischemia

5. _____ Collateral flow

Definitions

a. Occurring after a meal
b. Relating to or affecting the viscera
c. Lack of blood flow to the viscera
d. Relating to additional blood vessels that aid or add to circulation
e. Relating to internal organs or blood vessels in the abdominal cavity

ANATOMY AND PHYSIOLOGY REVIEW

IMAGE LABELING

Complete the labels in the images that follow.

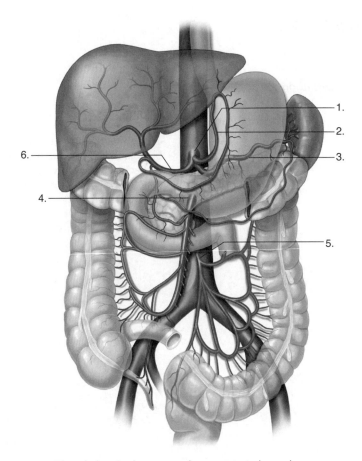

The abdominal aorta and mesenteric branches.

CHAPTER REVIEW

MULTIPLE CHOICE

Complete each question by circling the best answer.

1. What is the first major branch arising from the abdominal aorta?
   a. Superior mesenteric artery
   b. Celiac artery
   c. Inferior mesenteric artery
   d. Right renal artery

2. What is the most common indication for mesenteric artery duplex evaluation?
   a. Acute mesenteric ischemia
   b. Median arcuate ligament compression syndrome
   c. Chronic mesenteric ischemia
   d. Mesenteric artery aneurysms

3. How many splanchnic vessels are typically involved in atherosclerotic occlusive disease before a patient becomes symptomatic?
   a. 1
   b. 2
   c. 3
   d. 4

4. When does the abdominal pain many patients feel, which is associated with chronic mesenteric ischemia, typically occur?
   a. After eating
   b. In a fasting state
   c. Constantly (fasting and nonfasting)
   d. With aerobic exercise

5. Because of the abdominal pain indicated in the above question, patients often experience which of the following?
   a. Overeating and weight gain
   b. Fear of exercise
   c. Nausea and vomiting
   d. Fear of food and weight loss

6. Which of the following is one of the collateral systems that are present in the mesenteric vascular system?
   a. Pancreaticoduodenal arcade
   b. Arc of Riolan
   c. Internal iliac to inferior mesenteric artery connections
   d. All of the above

7. Most often, a replaced right hepatic artery originates from which vessel?
   a. Celiac artery
   b. Superior mesenteric artery
   c. Right renal artery
   d. Inferior mesenteric artery

8. With a patient in a fasting state, what should the superior mesenteric artery exhibit?
   a. High-resistance flow pattern
   b. Low-resistance flow pattern
   c. Mixed high- and low-resistance flow pattern
   d. Respiratory phasic flow pattern

9. Standard criteria for determining velocity thresholds for identifying stenosis in the celiac and superior mesenteric arteries were determined with the patient in what state?
   a. Fasting
   b. Postprandial
   c. Upright
   d. Pre- and postprandial

10. The term "seagull sign" is used to describe which of the following vessels?
    a. Superior mesenteric artery and its major branches
    b. Inferior mesenteric artery and its major branches
    c. Celiac, hepatic, and splenic arteries
    d. Left and right renal arteries

11. What should Doppler waveforms obtained from the celiac, splenic, and hepatic arteries demonstrate?
    a. High-resistance flow
    b. Mixed high- and low-resistance flow
    c. Prolonged systolic upstrokes
    d. Low-resistance flow

12. During a mesenteric artery evaluation, retrograde flow is noted in the common hepatic artery. What is this finding consistent with?
    a. Common hepatic artery stenosis
    b. Celiac artery occlusion
    c. Superior mesenteric artery stenosis
    d. Replaced right hepatic artery

13. Which of the following techniques can NOT be used to positively identify and differentiate the celiac and superior mesenteric vessels?

    a. Having the patient suspend breathing to reduce vessel movement

    b. Visualizing both the celiac and superior mesenteric arteries in the same image

    c. Visualizing aliasing with color flow in the superior mesenteric artery

    d. Documenting characteristic low-resistance flow in the celiac artery

14. Turning color flow imaging off can help identify which of the following?

    a. Arterial dissection

    b. Characterization of atherosclerotic plaque

    c. Stent placement within the vessel

    d. All of the above

15. During duplex evaluation of the mesenteric vessels, the SMA is noted to have velocities of 350 cm/s proximally with velocities of close to 300 cm/s in the midsegment. No spectral broadening or turbulence is noted. These findings are consistent with which of the following?

    a. Compensatory flow through the SMA likely due to occlusion of the celiac artery

    b. Significant stenosis of the SMA through its proximal and midsegments

    c. Occlusion of the SMA with reconstitution in the midsegment

    d. Normal SMA findings with normal velocities

16. Which of the following describes the velocity criteria for diagnosis of ≥70% in the celiac and superior mesenteric arteries?

    a. >275 cm/s PSV in the celiac and >200 cm/s PSV in the superior mesenteric artery

    b. >325 cm/s PSV in both the celiac and superior mesenteric arteries

    c. >200 cm/s PSV in the celiac and >275 cm/s PSB in the superior mesenteric artery

    d. >50 cm/s EDV in the celiac and >55 cm/s EDV in the superior mesenteric artery

17. Why may standard duplex ultrasound velocity criteria for mesenteric vessels NOT be accurate after treatment by stent placement?

    a. Velocities in treated vessels are considerably lower than standard criteria

    b. Velocities in treated vessels are typically higher than standard criteria

    c. Stented vessels are not well visualized on duplex scanning

    d. Stent struts artifactually decrease reflections, making Doppler signals inaccurate

18. What is transient compression of the celiac artery origin during exhalation, which is relieved by inhalation, characteristic of?

    a. Acute mesenteric ischemia

    b. Atherosclerotic disease at the celiac artery origin

    c. Compression of celiac artery from abdominal aortic aneurysm

    d. Median arcuate ligament compression syndrome

19. Visceral artery aneurysms are rare; however, the greatest incidence of aneurysms occurs in which of the following vessels?

    a. Splenic artery

    b. Common hepatic artery

    c. Celiac artery

    d. Superior mesenteric artery

20. What is the general role of the vascular laboratory in the diagnosis of acute mesenteric ischemia?

    a. Identification of the thrombus at the origin of the SMA

    b. No role due to the emergent nature of the illness

    c. Characterization of the stenosis and degree of narrowing

    d. Identification of the branch vessel in which embolus is likely to have occurred

FILL-IN-THE-BLANK

1. The celiac artery, the _____ branch of the abdominal aorta, is best visualized with the transducer oriented _____ and is located 1 to 2 cm below the _____. The superior mesenteric artery is best visualized with the transducer oriented _____ and originates from the _____ surface of the aorta 1 to 2 cm below the _____ artery.

2. The diagnosis of _____ mesenteric ischemia is difficult because the disorder is _____ and the symptoms are _____. It is often overlooked as the patient is worked up for _____, _____, _____, and _____ etiologies.

3. Only a small fraction of patients with
_____ mesenteric disease
develop true mesenteric _____
because of the rich _____
network. This network includes the superior and
inferior _____ arcade, the arc of
_____, and collaterals between
the internal _____ and inferior
_____ arteries.

4. Indications for duplex screening for chronic
mesenteric _____
include _____ pain
and _____ with
_____, presence of an
abdominal _____, and
_____ loss.

5. The classic symptom of mesenteric ischemia,
post_____ pain, results due to
insufficient _____ blood flow
following a _____ to support the
increased _____ demand required
to support _____ functions of
_____, _____,
and _____.

6. The most common anatomic anomaly in the
mesenteric system is a _____ right
_____ artery, originating from the
_____ _____
artery instead of the _____ artery.

7. When presenting to the vascular lab for mesenteric
vessel evaluation, it is critically important for
the patient to _____ for at
least 6 hours prior. This is necessary because
the _____ mesenteric artery
changes dramatically from _____
resistance to _____ and
_____ thresholds have been
established in this state.

8. When evaluating the mesenteric vessels
with Doppler, the sample volume should
be "_____" from the
_____ through the origin and
proximal segments of the _____,
_____ mesenteric
and _____ mesenteric
arteries in order to identify the highest
_____ _____
and _____
_____ velocities.

9. The term "seagull sign" refers to the sonographic
appearance of the _____ artery
and its branches, the _____
and _____ arteries. Normal
Doppler waveforms in these vessels demonstrate
a _____-resistance pattern with
_____ flow throughout systole
and _____.

10. The _____ mesenteric artery is
most easily identified in a _____
view by locating the aortic _____
and then scanning _____ 1 to
3 cm; this vessel typically originates from the
_____ aorta slightly to the
_____ of midline.

11. Asking the patient to _____
breathing can help to decrease
_____ of the mesenteric vessels,
thereby allowing positive _____
of vessels and improving Doppler
_____ accuracy.

12. In the presence of celiac artery
_____ or
_____, flow can be diverted
through the _____ artery, causing
_____ flow in the common
_____ artery.

13. In preparation for a duplex scan after mesenteric revascularization, it's important to review the _____ report. This report will detail the _____ of the proximal and distal _____, type of _____ graft or other intervention, and the graft _____.

14. When evaluating a mesenteric bypass graft, the Doppler exam should start with the _____ artery and continue through the proximal _____, _____ of the graft, the _____ anastomosis, and the _____ artery.

15. Increased velocities in the absence of _____ could be the result of _____ flow. A prominent _____ mesenteric artery, for example, may suggest _____ or stenosis of the _____ mesenteric artery with _____ through a meandering mesenteric artery.

16. The normal spectral Doppler waveform of the SMA demonstrates a sharp _____ upstroke with a _____ band of velocities with _____-resistance outflow characteristics. Peak systolic velocities are normally less than _____ cm/s with PSV above _____ cm/s consistent with a greater than _____% stenosis.

17. End-_____ velocities can also be used as thresholds for disease in the celiac and superior mesenteric arteries. This criteria states that velocity of _____ cm/s or greater is consistent with a greater than _____ %

stenosis in the celiac artery and greater than _____ cm/s in the superior mesenteric artery, also consistent with greater than _____% stenosis.

18. The _____ mesenteric artery does not have commonly accepted _____ criteria for diagnosis of stenosis. Instead, the general pattern of _____ velocity and post_____ _____ can be used to identify stenosis.

19. Studies completed in evaluation of stented visceral arteries conclude that SMA duplex velocity criteria of _____ vessels will likely _____ the prevalence of _____ or _____ disease after stenting.

20. An advantage of using duplex ultrasound to evaluate median _____ ligament _____ syndrome is that Doppler waveforms can be obtained during _____ as well as _____, thereby demonstrating the change in celiac artery _____ during the phases of the respiratory cycle.

21. Visceral artery aneurysms are _____ and are usually identified _____. The greatest incidence of visceral artery aneurysms occurs in the _____ artery and is more common in _____ than _____.

22. Causes of visceral artery dissections include _____, _____ dysplasia, _____ infection, _____,

connective _____

disorder, _____, and

_____-induced dissections.

23. Treatment of superior mesenteric artery

dissections includes _____

management with _____ or

more aggressive treatment with endovascular

_____ placement and

_____ procedures.

24. _____ mesenteric ischemia

can result from _____ to the

mesenteric arteries or _____ of an

artery with existing _____ disease.

25. Symptoms associated with acute mesenteric

_____ are typically described

as pain out of _____ to

_____ findings. Diagnosis must be

made quickly to avoid bowel _____

and high _____ rate.

SHORT ANSWER

1. What are the typical symptoms of chronic mesenteric ischemia? Describe the pathophysiological process that occurs to cause these symptoms.

2. List the current minimum requirements for image and Doppler waveform documentation for a mesenteric duplex exam.

3. What is the purpose of using a "test meal" when evaluating the mesenteric vessels?

IMAGE EVALUATION/PATHOLOGY

Review the images and answer the following questions.

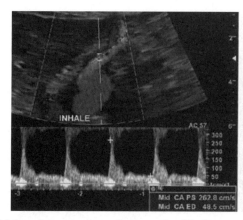 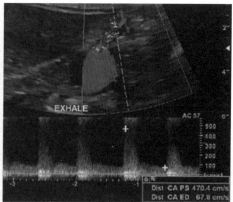

1. A 32-year-old female presents to the vascular lab for an abdominal bruit. The above images were taken during the exam of the abdominal aorta. Describe the findings present in the images.

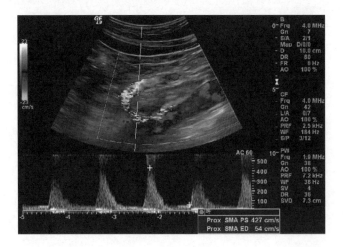

2. A 73-year-old female presents to the vascular lab with abdominal pain after eating and a recent history of weight loss. Duplex imaging of the abdominal aorta and its branches reveals the above images. Describe the findings. What other vessels should be evaluated and why?

CASE STUDY

Review the information and answer the following questions.

1. A 68-year-old female presents to the emergency room with acute onset of severe abdominal pain. Upon physical examination, nothing is found to be consistent with the amount of pain the patient is in. Based on this limited history, what should be suspected? What next steps should the patient undergo?

2. A 40-year-old multiparous female presents for abdominal duplex examination for suspicion of gallbladder disease. During this evaluation, an anechoic, circular mass is noted superior to the pancreas that appears to be in communication with the splenic artery. Color and spectral Doppler demonstrate flow within the mass. What should be suspected in this patient? What is the prognosis for this patient?

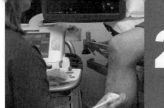

20 The Renal Vasculature

REVIEW OF GLOSSARY TERMS

MATCHING

Match the key terms with their definitions.

Key Terms

1. _____ Renal–aortic velocity ratio
2. _____ Poststenotic signal
3. _____ Renal medulla
4. _____ Renal hilum
5. _____ Renal ostium
6. _____ Renal sinus
7. _____ Renal cortex
8. _____ Renal parenchymal disease
9. _____ Renal artery stenosis
10. _____ Renal artery stent

Definitions

a. The central echogenic cavity of the kidney; contains the renal artery, renal vein, and collecting and lymphatic systems
b. Narrowing of the renal artery, most commonly as a result of atherosclerotic disease or medial fibromuscular dysplasia
c. A medical disorder affecting the tissue function of the kidneys
d. The peak systolic renal artery velocity divided by the peak systolic aortic velocity recorded at the level of the celiac and/or superior mesenteric arteries; used to identify flow-limiting renal artery stenosis
e. The area through which the renal artery, vein, and ureter enter the kidney
f. A tiny tube inserted into a stenotic renal artery at the time of arterial dilation; usually metallic mesh in structure; holds the artery open
g. A Doppler spectral waveform recorded immediately distal to a flow-reducing stenosis that exhibits decreased peak systolic velocity and disordered flow
h. The opening of the renal artery from the aortic wall
i. The middle area of the kidney lying between the sinus and the cortex; contains renal pyramids
j. The outermost area of the kidney tissue lying just beneath the renal capsule

ANATOMY AND PHYSIOLOGY REVIEW

IMAGE LABELING

Complete the labels in the images that follow.

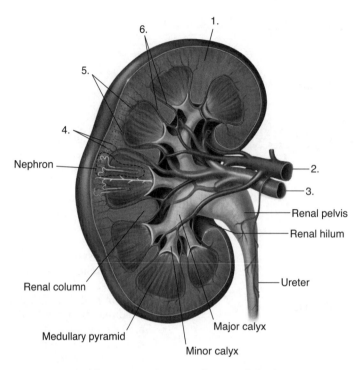

Nephron

Renal column

Medullary pyramid

Minor calyx

1.

6.

5.

4.

2.

3.

Renal pelvis

Renal hilum

Ureter

Major calyx

Diagram illustrating the vasculature of the kidneys.

CHAPTER REVIEW

MULTIPLE CHOICE

Complete each question by circling the best answer.

1. It is estimated that up to how many hypertensive patients have underlying renal artery disease?
   a. 50%
   b. 40%
   c. 6%
   d. 15%

2. Which of the following is NOT a limitation of contrast angiography?
   a. Detailed anatomic information
   b. Lack of hemodynamic information
   c. No identification of functional significance of renal artery disease
   d. Invasive with possible nephrotoxic contrast

3. Which of the following is true regarding duplex ultrasound assessment of the renal vasculature?
   a. Provides anatomic information
   b. Provides hemodynamic information
   c. Painless and noninvasive
   d. All of the above

4. What is the normal length measurement of the kidney?
   a. 4 to 5 cm
   b. 8 to 13 cm
   c. 10 to 15 cm
   d. 5 to 7 cm

5. What are kidneys that are joined at the lower poles by an isthmus of tissue, which lies anterior to the aorta, known as?
   a. Ectopic kidneys
   b. Cross-fused kidneys
   c. Horseshoe kidneys
   d. Junctional kidneys

6. Why is the renal sinus is normally brightly echogenic on a sonographic image?
   a. Lymphatic vessel location
   b. Fat and fibrous tissue in the sinus
   c. Increased blood flow in the area
   d. Fluid from the collecting system

7. What are the triangular-shaped structures within the inner portion of the kidney that carry urine from the cortex to the renal pelvis?
   a. Nephrons
   b. Columns of Bertin
   c. Renal pyramids
   d. Renal calyces

8. The right renal artery initially courses _____ from the aorta, then passes _____ to the inferior vena cava.
   a. Posterolateral, anterior
   b. Posterior, superior
   c. Anterolateral, laterally
   d. Anterolateral, posterior

9. Which of the following vessels courses anterior to the aorta but posterior to the superior mesenteric artery and anterior to both renal arteries?
   a. Splenic vein
   b. Right renal vein
   c. Left renal vein
   d. Inferior mesenteric vein

10. Atherosclerotic disease in the renal artery typically occurs in which of the following renal artery segments?
    a. Origin to proximal third
    b. Distal renal artery just before entering the kidney
    c. Mid- to distal segment
    d. Interlobar arteries within the renal parenchyma

11. Which of the following patients would be suspected of fibromuscular dysplasia in the renal artery?
    a. An 85-year-old diabetic male
    b. A 66-year-old female with a history of well-controlled hypertension and smoking
    c. A 25-year-old male with chronic asthma
    d. A 32-year-old female with poorly controlled hypertension

12. What is the most appropriate transducer for use in the evaluation of the renal arteries?
    a. 7 to 10 MHz straight linear
    b. 2 to 5 MHz curved linear
    c. 1 to 2 MHz vector array
    d. 5 to 8 MHz phased sector array

13. A spectral Doppler waveform with peak systolic velocity is needed from the aorta at which level for use in the renal–aortic ratio?
    a. Proximal, at the level of the celiac and superior mesenteric arteries
    b. Mid-, at the level of the renal arteries
    c. Distal, at the level of the inferior mesenteric artery
    d. Distal, at the level of the common iliac bifurcation

14. To identify the renal artery ostia, an image is obtained from which location?
    a. Transverse, at the level of the celiac artery
    b. Sagittal, at the level of the celiac artery
    c. Transverse, slightly inferior to the superior mesenteric artery
    d. Sagittal, slightly superior to the left renal vein

15. Which of the following is an ultrasound modality that has a low-angle dependence that may be helpful in identifying duplicate renal arteries?
    a. Color flow Doppler
    b. Power Doppler
    c. Spectral Doppler
    d. Pulse inversion Doppler

16. Flow patterns within the kidney parenchyma are typically obtained with a spectral Doppler using which angle of insonation?
    a. 60 degrees
    b. 90 degrees
    c. 0 degrees
    d. 45 degrees

17. When comparing renal length from side to side, how much of a difference suggests compromised flow in the smaller kidney?
    a. 1 cm
    b. 2 mm
    c. 3 mm
    d. 3 cm

18. Which of the following describe normal spectral Doppler waveform characteristics in the renal artery?
    a. High-resistance, minimal diastolic flow with velocities in the range of 90 to 120 cm/s
    b. Low-resistance, high-diastolic flow with velocities in the range of 90 to 120 cm/sec
    c. Low-resistance, minimal diastolic flow with velocities in the range of 10 to 120 cm/s
    d. High-resistance, high-diastolic flow with velocities in the range of 50 to 70 cm/s

19. A patient presents to the vascular laboratory for a renal artery duplex evaluation. During the exam, velocities in the right renal artery origin reach 175 cm/s with no evidence of poststenotic turbulence. Velocities on the left were 100 cm/s. What do these findings suggest?
    a. Right renal artery stenosis <60%
    b. Left renal artery stenosis <60%
    c. Right renal artery stenosis >60%
    d. Left renal artery stenosis >60%

20. Which of the following spectral Doppler waveform changes will occur distal to the stenosis with hemodynamically significant stenosis of the renal artery?
    a. Delayed systolic upstroke
    b. Loss of compliance peak
    c. Decreased peak systolic velocity
    d. Increased peak systolic velocity

21. Which of the following findings within the kidney are consistent with renal artery occlusion?
    a. Kidney length of >10 cm, velocities less than 10 cm/s in the renal cortex
    b. Kidney length of <9 cm, velocities less than 10 cm/s in the renal cortex
    c. Kidney length >13 cm with no detectable flow within the renal parenchyma
    d. Kidney length <9 cm, velocities greater than 20 cm/s in the renal cortex

22. A patient presents to the vascular lab with suspected acute tubular necrosis. Which of the following findings on the renal artery duplex exam would be consistent with this condition?
    a. Renal artery velocities >180 cm/s, EDR of 0.35
    b. Renal artery velocities >180 cm/s, RI of 0.6
    c. Renal artery velocities of 70 cm/s, EDR of 0.19
    d. Renal artery velocities of 70 cm/s, RI of 0.5

23. What is measured to determine acceleration time?
    a. Onset of systole to the early systolic peak
    b. Onset of systole to the end of diastole
    c. Onset of diastole to the early systolic peak
    d. End diastole to end systole

24. During a renal artery duplex exam, the following were found: proximal aorta velocities of 100 mc/s, proximal right renal artery velocity of 200 cm/s, and proximal left renal artery velocities of 400 cm/s. Which of the following describes these findings?
    a. Right RAR = 2.0, <60% stenosis; Left RAR = 0.4, <60% stenosis
    b. Right RAR = 0.2, >60% stenosis, Left RAR = 0.4, >60% stenosis
    c. Right RAR = 2.0, <60% stenosis; Left RAR = 4.0, >60% stenosis
    d. Right RAR = 0.2, >60% stenosis; Left RAR = 4.0, <60% stenosis

25. In the above question, for which renal artery would you expect to see poststenotic turbulence?
    a. Right
    b. Left
    c. Both
    d. Neither

26. Which of the following may result in misinterpretation of the hilar acceleration time?
    a. Elevated renovascular resistance
    b. Systemic arterial stiffness
    c. Renal artery stenosis in the 60% to 79% range
    d. All of the above

27. Under which conditions is the renal-to-aortic ratio likely inaccurate?
    a. The abdominal aortic velocities are between 75 and 90 cm/s
    b. The abdominal aortic velocities are over 100 cm/s or below 40 cm/s
    c. The renal artery velocities exceed 300 cm/s
    d. The renal artery velocities are below 100 cm/s

28. During renal duplex evaluation, the left renal vein near the hilum is noted to have continuous, nonphasic low-velocity flow. What do these findings suggest?
    a. Renal artery stenosis
    b. Normal renal vein findings
    c. Proximal renal vein thrombosis
    d. Distal renal vein thrombosis

29. A patient presents to the vascular lab for follow-up after renal artery stent placement. Velocities within the distal segment of the stent reach 250 cm/s. At other follow-ups at 6 and 12 months, velocities in the distal stent remain 250 cm/s. What are these findings consistent with?

    a. Increased velocity due to size mismatch from the stent to native vessel

    b. Fixed stenosis at the distal end of the stent

    c. Kinking of the stent, creating artificially elevated velocities

    d. Stent collapse and failure

30. Which of the following represents renal duplex findings that demonstrate a high risk for renal atrophy and likely unsuccessful renal revascularization?

    a. Renal artery PSV <400 cm/s and cortical EDV >10 cm/s

    b. Renal artery PSV >400 cm/s and cortical EDV <5 cm/s

    c. Renal artery PSV >160 cm/s and cortical EDV <10 cm/s

    d. Renal artery PSV >200 cm/s and cortical EDV <5 cm/s

FILL-IN-THE-BLANK

1. Renal artery stenosis should be suspected in adults with _____ onset of chronic _____; azotemia, which is induced by _____- _____ enzyme inhibitor; unexplained renal _____; or pulmonary _____.

2. In most patients, renal artery disease is _____ with treatment providing control of or cure for _____ hypertension, retention of _____ mass, and _____ of renal function in patients with chronic renal _____.

3. Because of the _____ of the contrast agents, computed tomography _____ is often reserved for use as secondary _____ study.

4. The kidneys are located _____ in the dorsal abdominal cavity between the _____ thoracic and _____ lumbar vertebrae.

5. The four main areas of the kidneys identified for sonographic interrogation are the renal _____, where the artery enters and the vein and ureter exit; the renal _____, which contains the artery, vein, and collecting system; the _____, which contains the renal pyramids; and the _____, where urine is produced.

6. The renal arteries can be identified approximately _____ cm below the _____ plane, with the left renal artery slightly more _____ than the right.

7. The right renal vein has a _____ course, whereas the left renal vein courses _____ to the aorta just below the origin of the _____ _____ artery.

8. The most common cause of renovascular disease is _____ renal artery stenosis, which occurs more commonly in _____ and elderly patients with _____, coronary or peripheral arterial disease, hyperlipidemia, or _____.

9. The second most common curable cause of renovascular disease is medial _____ _____, which occurs most commonly in _____ aged _____ years.

10. Positions that may be used in order to visualize the entire renal artery as well as the kidney include _____ in reverse Trendelenberg, right or left _____ _____, and possibly _____ with the patient's mid-section flexed over a pillow.

11. A spectral Doppler signal should be obtained from the abdominal aorta at the level of the _____ and _____ _____ arteries for use in calculation of the _____-_____ velocity ratio.

12. From a midline abdominal approach, the _____ to _____-segments of the renal arteries may be visualized. Using this approach, the Doppler sample _____ can be walked from the _____ lumen through the renal _____ in order to rule out orificial renal artery stenosis.

13. Duplicate renal arteries may be detected on a _____, _____ image of the aorta. Using _____ Doppler is valuable in identifying these small vessels because of its lower _____ dependence and sensitivity to _____-flow states.

14. In addition to evaluation of the renal vasculature, the parenchyma of the kidney should be examined for _____ thinning, renal _____, masses, _____, or _____.

15. Kidney _____ is important to document as a shortened kidney is suggestive of a _____-limiting renal artery lesion. A difference in renal length greater than _____ cm suggests compromised flow on the side with the _____ kidney.

16. In the presence of renal vein _____, renal artery waveforms demonstrate _____, _____ diastolic flow components.

17. The proximal aorta demonstrates rapid systolic _____ and forward _____ flow, whereas the distal abdominal aorta demonstrates a _____ flow pattern that reflects the elevated vascular _____ of the lower extremities.

18. The spectral Doppler waveform from the normal renal artery is characterized by rapid _____ upstroke, a slightly _____ peak, and forward _____ flow. An early _____ or _____ peak is often seen on the upstroke to systole.

19. A flow-reducing stenosis of the renal artery demonstrates velocities greater than _____ cm/s poststenotic _____. When the degree of narrowing exceeds _____%, the systolic upstroke is _____, the _____ peak is lost, and the PSV will _____ distally.

20. With chronic renal artery _____, the PSV in the cortex will be less than _____ cm/s and pole-to-pole _____ of the kidney will be less than _____ cm.

21. Normal flow in the parenchyma of the kidney demonstrates _____ high _____ flow throughout all segments of the kidney; often, this flow is _____% to _____% of the systolic velocity. When parenchymal disease is present, increased renovascular _____ is demonstrated throughout the kidney, characterized by _____ diastolic flow.

22. Indirect renal _____ evaluations use _____ index or time to provide assessment of renal artery _____. The theory of this method is that delayed systolic _____ will result _____ to a significant stenosis.

23. Limitations of the indirect assessment of renal artery stenosis include normal acceleration time in patients with elevated _____ resistance, normal Doppler waveform contour in patients with _____% stenosis or _____ renal arteries, and damped intrarenal spectral waveforms in patients with aortic _____ or _____.

24. Current diagnostic criteria for identification of renal artery stenosis are based on the _____–_____ ratio, which is the ratio of the _____ artery PSV to the _____ PSV. A hemodynamically significant stenosis in the renal artery will result in a ratio greater than _____.

25. When evaluating a stented renal artery, slight velocity _____ are typically identified, making identification of restenosis difficult. Recent research suggests that using a peak systolic velocity of greater than _____ cm/s and a _____–aortic ratio of greater than _____ will result in a determination of in-stent _____.

SHORT ANSWER

1. Describe the appropriate patient preparation and positioning for a renal artery duplex examination.

2. Describe the imaging and Doppler techniques used to evaluate the entire length of the renal arteries.

3. List the diagnostic criteria used to determine renal artery stenosis and intrinsic renal parenchymal disease. What are the limitations of these criteria?

IMAGE EVALUATION/PATHOLOGY

Review the images and answer the following questions.

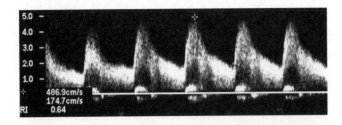

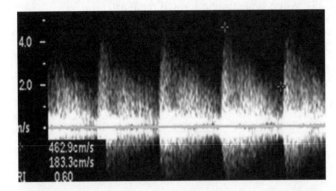

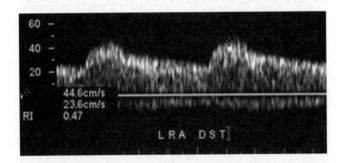

1. These spectral Doppler waveforms were taken from the left renal artery origin, proximal and distal segment, respectively. What do these images suggest?

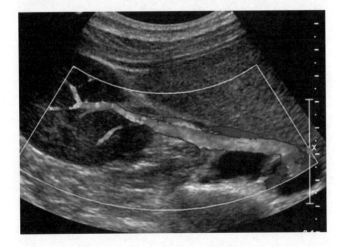

2. This image demonstrates the right renal artery and inferior vena cava. What anomaly is present?

CASE STUDY

Review the information and answer the following questions.

1. A 68-year-old male with chronic hypertension presents to the vascular laboratory for renal artery duplex evaluation. The patient's history also includes diabetes, hyperlipidemia, angina, and smoking. During the renal artery duplex exam, the following was found: right renal artery PSV 325 cm/s and EDV 140 cm/s with turbulence noted just past the origin; left renal artery of 185 cm/s and EDV 80 cm/s, no turbulence is noted; proximal aorta PSV 85 cm/s. In the renal hila, acceleration times are 105 ms on the right and 80 ms on the left. What do these findings suggest?

2. A 37-year-old female presents to the vascular lab with uncontrolled hypertension for renal artery duplex examination. What disease process should be suspected in this patient? What should the vascular technologist be on the lookout for during a renal artery duplex examination?

3. An 82-year-old female presents to the vascular laboratory with elevated serum creatinine and blood urea nitrogen levels. During renal artery duplex examination, velocities from the renal arteries remain within normal limits. Upon evaluation of the renal parenchyma, peak systolic velocities are 25 cm/s with end-diastolic velocities of 6 cm/s, bilaterally. What is the resistive index and diastolic-to-systolic ratio in the kidneys? What do these findings suggest?

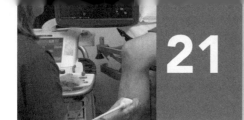

21 The Inferior Vena Cava and Iliac Veins

REVIEW OF GLOSSARY TERMS

MATCHING

Match the key terms with their definitions.

Key Terms

1. __C__ Retroperitoneum
2. __E__ Inferior vena cava filter
3. __A__ Pulmonary embolus
4. __D__ Thrombosis
5. __B__ Confluence

Definitions

a. The obstruction of the pulmonary arteries, usually from detached fragments of a blood clot that travels from the lower extremity

b. The union of two or more veins to form a larger vein; the equivalent of a bifurcation in the arterial system

c. The space between the abdominal cavity and the muscles and bones of the posterior abdominal wall

d. Partial or complete occlusion of a blood vessel due to clot

e. A typically cone-shaped medical device designed to prevent pulmonary embolism

ANATOMY AND PHYSIOLOGY REVIEW

IMAGE LABELING

Complete the labels in the image that follows.

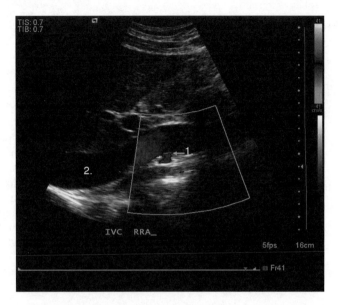

Sagittal image through the mid-abdomen.

CHAPTER REVIEW

MULTIPLE CHOICE

Complete each question by circling the best answer.

1. What is the external iliac vein a continuation of?
   a. Common iliac vein
   b. Great saphenous vein
   c. Common femoral vein
   d. Inferior vena cava

2. In well-hydrated patients, what is the mean diameter of the inferior vena cava at the level of the renal veins?
   a. 17 to 20 mm
   b. 10 to 15 mm
   c. 2 to 3 cm
   d. 3 to 5 cm

3. Where does the left-sided IVC in a duplicate system typically terminate?
   a. Splenic vein
   b. Right renal vein
   c. Superior mesenteric vein
   d. Left renal vein

4. Upon ultrasound examination, the hepatic veins are noted to drain directly into the right atrium. What does this finding suggest?
   a. Normal findings in the hepatic veins
   b. Congenital absence of the inferior vena cava
   c. Membranous obstruction of the intrahepatic IVC
   d. Duplicate inferior vena cava syndrome

5. Which of the following is an impediment to visualizing the inferior vena cava?
   a. Overlying bowel gas
   b. Morbid obesity
   c. Open abdominal wounds
   d. All of the above

6. While applying pressure to the patient's abdomen may disperse bowel gas to make visualization of the IVC easier, why must care be taken?
   a. Excessive force can compress the IVC
   b. Gentle pressure may result in bruising of the patient
   c. Excessive force may result in compression of the aorta
   d. Gentle pressure can create a stenosis in the IVC

7. The inferior vena cava should be evaluated in both sagittal and transverse from the diaphragm to what level?
   a. The renal veins
   b. The confluence of the common iliac veins
   c. The hepatic veins
   d. Mid-abdomen and lumbar veins

8. From a coronal plane in the left lateral decubitus position, what landmark can be used to identify the confluence of the common iliac veins to create the IVC?
   a. Superior pole of the right kidney
   b. Left lobe of the liver
   c. Inferior pole of the right kidney
   d. Inferior pole of the left kidney

9. Which of the following describes normal IVC and iliac vein imaging characteristics?
   a. Thin, echogenic walls with anechoic lumens
   b. Thin, hypoechoic walls with hyperechoic lumens
   c. Thick, muscular walls that are hypoechoic with hyperechoic lumens
   d. Anechoic walls with hypoechoic lumens

10. What is the most common pathologic finding in the IVC and iliac veins?
    a. Tumor extension from renal cell carcinoma
    b. Thrombus extension from deep venous thrombosis in the legs
    c. Isolated thrombosis of the IVC
    d. Venous dissection through the iliac veins

11. Newly formed thrombus appears virtually _____, whereas more advanced thrombus appears _____.
    a. Hyperechoic, anechoic
    b. Hyperechoic, hypoechoic
    c. Hypoechoic, hypoechoic
    d. Anechoic, hyperechoic

12. What do intraluminal tumors in the inferior vena cava most commonly arise from?
    a. Pancreatic carcinoma
    b. Colon carcinoma
    c. Renal carcinoma
    d. Bladder carcinoma

13. One way that intraluminal tumors can be distinguished from thrombosis is that tumors demonstrate which of the following?
    a. Flow within the mass
    b. Anechoic texture
    c. Lack of flow in the mass
    d. Change in echogenicity over time

14. Which of the following Doppler modes would best be able to detect the slow-flow states that are typically seen in the inferior vena cava and iliac veins?
    a. Color Doppler
    b. Power Doppler
    c. Spectral Doppler
    d. CW Doppler

15. Color flow Doppler can be particular useful in identifying tissue bruits and pulsatile flow in the presence of which of the following?
    a. Filter perforation
    b. Deep venous thrombosis
    c. Tumor extension
    d. Aortocaval fistula

16. During spectral Doppler analysis of the iliac system, continuous flow is noted in the common iliac veins bilaterally. What is this finding consistent with?
    a. Obstruction in the common iliac veins
    b. Obstruction in the common femoral veins
    c. Obstruction in the inferior vena cava
    d. Normal findings in the common iliac veins

17. What is the condition that occurs when the left common iliac vein is compressed between the overlying right common iliac artery and underlying vertebral body known as?
    a. May-Thurner syndrome
    b. Raynaud's syndrome
    c. Arcuate ligament syndrome
    d. Paget-Schroetter syndrome

18. What is filter placement in the inferior vena cava designed to prevent?
    a. Thrombus extension from the lower extremities
    b. Pulmonary embolus
    c. Thrombus extension from the intrahepatic inferior vena cava
    d. Tumor extension from the renal veins

19. Which of the following is a dependable marker for ultrasound identification of the level of the renal veins for IVC filter placement?
    a. Superior mesenteric artery
    b. Superior mesenteric vein
    c. Left renal vein
    d. Right renal artery

20. On sonographic evaluation, which of the following describes the appearance of an IVC filter?
    a. Hypoechoic, circular rings within the IVC lumen
    b. Hyperechoic, circular rings within the IVC lumen
    c. Echogenic lines that converge to a point
    d. Hypoechoic lines that converge to a point

FILL-IN-THE-BLANK

1. The _____ iliac veins drain the pelvic _____ and musculature and join the _____ iliac veins at the level of the _____ joints to form the _____ iliac veins.

2. The inferior vena cava begins at the junction of the right and left _____ iliac veins at the level of the _____ lumbar vertebra and ascends in the retroperitoneum to the _____ of the abdominal aorta.

3. _____ causes a collapse of the IVC, making it difficult to visualize, whereas _____ heart failure may cause _____ cava.

4. With _____ obstruction of the intrahepatic IVC, a _____ septum may be visualized in the IVC, and flow in the distal hepatic veins is _____ and _____.

5. When evaluating the IVC, the height of the bed should be adjusted so that the level of the patient's _____ is slightly lower than the sonographer's _____ to ergonomically apply pressure.

6. A complete exam of the IVC requires a _____ and _____ survey from the _____ to the confluence of the _____ iliac veins.

7. Landmarks that can be used to identify the IVC in a longitudinal plane include the _____, which lies to the left of the IVC and the _____, which lies anterior to the IVC.

8. The _____ plane may offer better imaging of the _____ IVC and confluence of the common _____ veins, using the _____ pole of the _____ kidney as a landmark.

9. When evaluating the iliac veins, the patient should be positioned _____ with the bed in a reverse _____ position.

10. _____ iliac veins can often be identified by following the _____ femoral vein from the groin into the pelvis. Due to its deep location, the _____ iliac vein is often difficult to visualize.

11. The normal IVC and iliac veins have _____, muscular walls with _____ lumens. With quiet _____, the _____ of the IVC may appear to change with the phasic changes in _____ pressure produced during respiration.

12. In the presence of thrombosis, grayscale imaging may reveal a _____ IVC or iliac vein with _____ material within the lumen. Acute thrombus may appear virtually _____ on gray scale; therefore, _____ and _____ Doppler are important to the examination.

13. Thrombus that does completely _____ flow may only be detected by _____ imaging demonstrating _____-floating echogenic material in the IVC or iliac vein _____.

14. Intraluminal tumor extension into the IVC typically appears as _____ material within the lumen with _____ within the mass of color flow imaging.

15. _____ tumors may completely or partially _____ the IVC or iliac veins, resulting in _____ collateral veins and _____ of the distal IVC and iliac veins.

16. An IVC _____ is used to protect patients from pulmonary _____ and is typically placed just _____ to the _____ veins.

17. _____ material found within and around an IVC filter represents trapped _____ and should be considered an _____ finding.

18. Normally, the _____ IVC demonstrates a _____ waveform pattern due to its proximity to the _____, whereas the distal IVC and iliac veins demonstrate respiratory _____.

19. Unlike in the lower extremity veins, the iliac veins cannot be evaluated with transducer _____ maneuvers; therefore, _____ Doppler becomes important in detecting iliac vein _____.

20. When evaluating the iliac veins with spectral Doppler, loss of _____ phasicity and inability to _____ with distal thigh compression indicate iliac vein _____.

21. Iliac vein _____ syndrome occurs when the _____ common iliac vein is compressed between

the overlying _____ common iliac artery. It is also known as _____-_____ syndrome and commonly presents as left _____ deep venous thrombosis.

22. _____ flow without respiratory _____ distal to iliac vein compression and _____ flow velocity at the point of compression are signs of iliac vein compression syndrome.

23. When using duplex ultrasound for guidance for IVC filter placement, the _____ renal _____ can be used as a marker to determine the level of the _____ veins, which the filter must be placed _____ to.

24. Rarely, an IVC filter may _____ the IVC, causing a _____, which can be seen on ultrasound imaging.

25. Benefits of ultrasound guidance for filter placement include performance of the procedure at _____, lack of exposure to _____, and no required use of intravenous _____.

SHORT ANSWER

1. What are the tributaries that drain into the inferior vena cava?

2. List the required images for an ultrasound examination of the inferior vena cava and iliac veins.

IMAGE EVALUATION/PATHOLOGY

Review the images and answer the following questions.

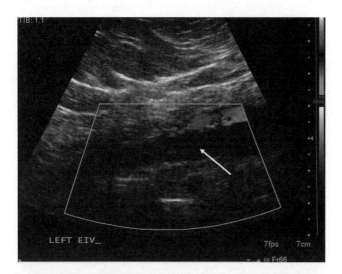

1. Describe the findings in this image. What additional information would aid in the diagnosis?

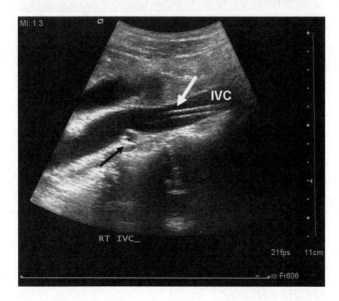

2. What is demonstrated in this image, indicated by the white arrow? What is its purpose?

3. What is the black arrow pointing to and why is this structure important?

CASE STUDY

Review the information and answer the following questions.

1. A 57-year-old female presents with bilateral lower extremity swelling. The patient has a history of renal cell carcinoma. What should the vascular technologist be concerned about in this patient?

2. During inferior vena cava and iliac vein ultrasound evaluation, a thrombus is noted in the right external iliac vein. Describe the spectral Doppler findings in the following vessels, including responses to distal augmentation maneuvers.

   a. Right common femoral vein

   b. Right common iliac vein

   c. Inferior vena cava

   d. Left common iliac vein

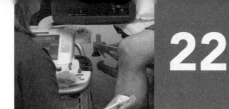

22 The Hepatoportal System

REVIEW OF GLOSSARY TERMS

MATCHING

Match the key terms with their definitions.

Key Terms

1. _____ Hepatopetal

2. _____ Hepatofugal

3. _____ Portal hypertension

4. _____ Budd-Chiari syndrome

5. _____ Ascites

Definitions

a. An accumulation of fluid within the peritoneal cavity
b. Elevated pressure within the portal vein
c. Hepatic vein thrombosis
d. Toward the liver, usually referring to normal direction of portal vein flow
e. Away from the liver

ANATOMY AND PHYSIOLOGY REVIEW

IMAGE LABELING

Complete the labels in the images that follow.

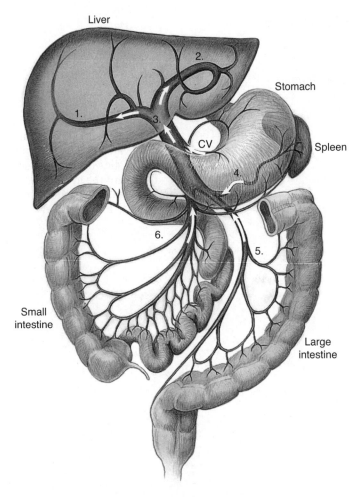

Vessels of the portal venous system.

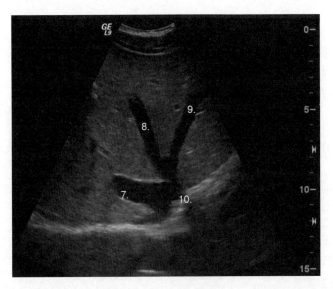

Vessels within the liver.

CHAPTER REVIEW

MULTIPLE CHOICE

Complete each question by circling the best answer.

1. The portal vein supplies approximately what percentage of blood into the liver?
   a. 30%
   b. 50%
   c. 70%
   d. 100%

2. What is the transverse fissure on the visceral surface of the liver between the caudate and quadrate lobes called?
   a. Main lobar fissure
   b. Porta hepatis
   c. Ligamentum venosum
   d. Falciform ligament

3. Which of the following describes the portal veins within the liver?
   a. Thin, invisible walls; course between the liver segments
   b. Thin, invisible walls; course within the liver segments
   c. Thick, bright walls; course between the liver segments
   d. Thick, bright walls; course within the liver segments

4. Which landmark identifies the start of the proper hepatic artery from the common hepatic artery?
   a. Gastroduodenal artery
   b. Splenic artery
   c. Superior mesenteric artery
   d. Portal vein

5. Which of the following patient positions offers excellent visualization of the porta hepatis?
   a. Transverse epigastric
   b. Transverse right costal
   c. Right coronal oblique
   d. Left coronal oblique

6. At which location should the portal vein diameter be measured?
   a. Just inside the liver before it branches into the right and left portal vein
   b. Where it crosses the inferior vena cava
   c. At the splenic–superior mesenteric vein confluence
   d. Where it crosses the aorta

7. What is normal portal vein diameter with quiet respiration?
   a. ≤13 mm
   b. >16 mm
   c. ≥13 mm
   d. ≤13 cm

8. What is an increase in caliber of less than 20% in the splenic vein during deep inspiration indicative of?
   a. Splenic vein thrombosis
   b. Budd-Chiari syndrome
   c. Portal hypertension
   d. Congestive heart failure

9. What increases blood flow within the portal, splenic, and superior mesenteric veins?
   a. Inspiration and ingestion of food
   b. Inspiration and exercise
   c. Expiration and exercise
   d. Expiration and ingestion of food

10. When assessing hepatic vein flow, the S and D wave should show blood flow toward which organ?
    a. Liver
    b. Heart
    c. Spleen
    d. Small intestine

11. What is a normal resistive index in the hepatic artery?
    a. 0.2 to 0.4
    b. 0.8 to 1.0
    c. 0.5 to 0.7
    d. 1.3 to 1.5

12. What is the most common etiology for portal hypertension in North America?
    a. Portal vein thrombosis
    b. Budd-Chiari syndrome
    c. Congestive heart failure
    d. Cirrhosis

13. What is the primary complication of portal hypertension?
    a. Portal vein thrombosis
    b. Gastrointestinal bleeding
    c. Hepatic vein thrombosis
    d. Splenomegaly

14. Which of the following is NOT a duplex sonographic finding associated with portal hypertension?

    a. Increased portal vein diameter

    b. Decreased or absent respiratory variation in portal and splenic veins

    c. Hepatopetal flow in the portal and splenic veins

    d. Portosystemic collaterals (varices)

15. What is the most common portosystemic collateral shunt in the presence of portal hypertension?

    a. Recanalized paraumbilical vein

    b. Splenorenal veins

    c. Gallbladder varices

    d. Coronary–gastroesophageal veins

16. Which of the following is a treatment of portal hypertension that involves jugular vein cannulation with stent placement in the liver?

    a. Mesocaval shunt

    b. Splenorenal shunt

    c. TIPS

    d. PVTS

17. Which of the following is NOT a normal finding in a transjugular portosystemic shunt?

    a. Hepatofugal flow in the main portal vein

    b. Velocities within the stent in the range of 90 to 190 cm/s

    c. Hepatofugal flow in intrahepatic portal veins beyond the site of stent connection

    d. Increased flow velocities in the splenic vein

18. Upon duplex evaluation of the portal system, the vascular technologists visualize increased portal vein caliber with no detectable flow by color, power, and spectral Doppler. Increased hepatic arterial flow is also documented. What are these findings consistent with?

    a. Portal hypertension

    b. Budd-Chiari syndrome

    c. Cirrhosis

    d. Portal vein thrombosis

19. Besides inferior vena cava dilatation, what distinct finding helps differentiate between congestive heart failure and portal hypertension?

    a. Increased pulsatility in the portal veins only

    b. Increased pulsatility in the hepatic veins only

    c. Increased pulsatility in both the portal and hepatic veins

    d. Decreased pulsatility in the hepatic veins only

20. Which of the following is NOT a sonographic finding in Budd-Chiari syndrome?

    a. Dilatation of the IVC with intraluminal echoes

    b. Pulsatile, phasic flow in nonoccluded portions of the hepatic veins

    c. Enlarged caudate lobe

    d. Ascites and hepatomegaly

FILL-IN-THE-BLANK

1. The main portal vein begins at the junction of the _____ vein and the

   _____ _____

   vein and lies _____ to the inferior

   vena cava.

2. After entering the liver through the

   _____ _____,

   the main portal vein branches into the right

   and left portal veins. The right portal vein then

   branches into _____ and

   _____ segments and the left

   portal vein branches into _____

   and _____ segments.

3. Hepatic veins drain the liver into the

   _____ _____

   _____, run

   _____ the lobes of the liver,

   and increase in _____ as they

   approach the _____.

4. Using the transverse epigastric plane, angling

   the transducer cephalad provides visualization

   of the _____ venous

   _____, whereas angling

   the transducer caudally allows visualization

   of the _____ vein and

   _____ confluence.

5. While performing a portal venous duplex

   exam, the liver should be examined

   for _____ and

_____, the spleen evaluated for _____, and the abdominal cavity for the presence of _____.

6. Spectral Doppler waveforms and velocity measurements should be documented from the _____, right, and left _____ veins; right, middle, and left _____ veins; splenic and _____ mesenteric veins; inferior vena cava; and _____ artery.

7. Using a higher frequency transducer during portal venous duplex exam can allow for better imaging of anterior abdominal wall _____ and assessing the liver surface for _____.

8. Major limitations affecting the success of portal venous duplex exams include patient _____, diffuse _____ disease, _____, and bowel _____, as well as patients who are not able to vary their _____.

9. Portal vein diameters increase in patients with portal _____, _____ heart _____, constrictive _____, and portal vein _____.

10. Portal venous flow is normally directed _____ the liver with constant _____ flow throughout the _____ cycle. Mean flow velocities are _____ cm/sec.

11. Hepatic veins exhibit _____ waveforms that correspond to cyclic _____ changes within the heart. In contrast, portal veins demonstrate _____ waveforms.

12. Spectral Doppler waveforms from the hepatic artery demonstrate a _____ resistance pattern with _____ flow throughout the cardiac cycle. With ingestion of food, portal vein flow velocities _____, whereas hepatic artery velocities _____.

13. Inferior vena cava diameters range from _____ mm; however, this diameter depends on patient _____, right _____ pressure, and fluid _____ or heart _____.

14. Portal pressure, the gradient from the _____ _____ _____ and the portal vein should be between _____ mm Hg. Portal hypertension becomes _____ significant when this pressure gradient exceeds _____ mm Hg.

15. The most common etiology for portal hypertension in North America is _____. Until recently, the most common cause of this disorder was _____ abuse; however, now _____ infection accounts for a larger percentage of cases.

16. Causes of portal hypertension can be divided into three levels: _____ (inflow), _____ (liver sinusoids), and _____ (outflow).

17. Sonographic findings of portal hypertension include portal vein diameter greater than _____ mm, _____ flow in the portal vein, and _____ hepatic artery flow.

18. Detection of _____ collaterals is the most _____ finding of portal hypertension. Commonly seen collaterals include _____ vein, _____ vein, _____ veins, and _____ vein.

19. Imaging findings of an enlarged _____ artery with _____ velocity, _____ flow is referred to as _____.

20. Causes of arterial–portal fistulae include _____ trauma, iatrogenic trauma secondary to liver _____, transhepatic _____, and transhepatic _____ of the bile ducts or portal veins.

21. When evaluating a TIPS, velocities should be recorded from the _____ portal vein, portal vein end of the _____, _____-shunt, _____ vein end of the shunt, and the _____.

22. A TIPS _____ should be suspected if _____ material is observed within the stent and flow is _____ on color and spectral Doppler.

23. Etiologies of portal vein thrombosis include flow stasis secondary to _____, _____ processes, various _____ states, _____ intervention, abdominal _____, sepsis, and _____.

24. If portal vein thrombosis persists without lysis, development of _____ collateral veins develops. This condition is known as _____ _____.

25. Clinical features associated with hepatic vein thrombosis include _____ upper quadrant pain, _____, ascites, _____, and liver _____ abnormalities suggesting hepatocellular dysfunction.

SHORT ANSWER

1. List the indications for hepatoportal duplex ultrasound.

2. List the scanning planes that are commonly used in portal duplex exams and the structures that are best visualized from these approaches.

3. What are the normal findings in a well-functioning TIPS?

IMAGE EVALUATION/PATHOLOGY

Review the images and answer the following questions.

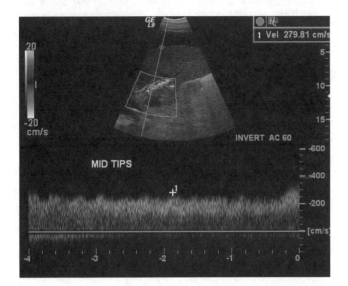

1. This Doppler waveform was taken from the mid-region of a TIPS. What are these findings consistent with?

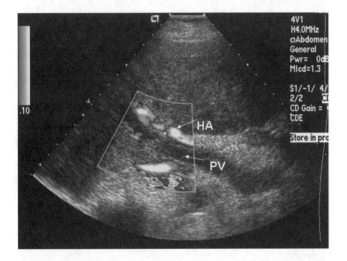

2. This image demonstrates power Doppler imaging at the porta hepatis. Describe the findings.

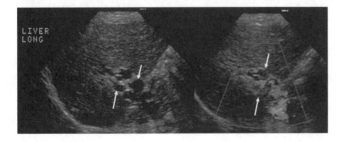

3. This image shows another view of the porta hepatis with color flow Doppler. Describe the findings.

CASE STUDY

Review the information and answer the following questions.

1. A 58-year-old male presents to the vascular lab for hepatoportal duplex exanimation with a history of alcoholism. What disorder should the vascular technologist be suspicious of in this patient and what are the sonographic findings associated with this disorder?

2. A 23-year-old female presents to the vascular lab for hepatoportal duplex examination. The patient presents with right upper quadrant pain, jaundice, ascites, and hepatomegaly and has a history of oral contraceptive use. What disorder should the vascular technologist expect and what are the sonographic findings of this disorder?

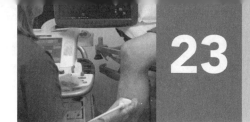

23 Evaluation of Kidney and Liver Transplants

REVIEW OF GLOSSARY TERMS

MATCHING

Match the key terms with their definitions.

Key Terms

1. _____ Allograft

2. _____ Orthotopic transplant

3. _____ Transplant rejection

4. _____ Immunosuppression drugs

5. _____ Arteriovenous fistula

6. _____ Pseudoaneurysm

Definition

a. The failure of a transplant occurring secondary to the formation of antidonor antibodies by the recipient. It can lead to loss of the transplant.

b. A connection between an artery and a vein, usually posttraumatic in origin.

c. Drugs used to inhibit the body's formation of antibodies to the allograft.

d. Develops secondary to a tear in the arterial wall allowing extravasation of blood from the arterial lumen, which is contained by a compacted rim of surrounding soft tissue.

e. A transplant that is placed in the same anatomic location as the native organ.

f. Any tissue transplanted from one human to another human

CHAPTER REVIEW

MULTIPLE CHOICE

Complete each question by circling the best answer.

1. Which of the following is NOT a symptom of graft failure?
   a. Elevated red blood count
   b. Fever and chills
   c. Elevated serum creatinine level
   d. Pain and tenderness

2. Where are kidney transplants most frequently placed?
   a. Normal kidney position
   b. Right iliac fossa position
   c. Left iliac fossa position
   d. Right posterior position

3. In a DD transplant, which vessel anastomosis is performed?
   a. Donor aortic wall and recipient external iliac artery
   b. Donor aortic wall and recipient internal iliac artery
   c. Recipient renal artery and donor external iliac artery
   d. Recipient external iliac artery and donor main renal artery

4. Which of the following is a renal transplant complication that is relatively common in the postsurgical period?
   a. Superinfection
   b. Urinoma
   c. Lymphocele
   d. Ureteral occlusion

5. What is the optimal time frame to perform a baseline sonogram in renal transplant patient?
   a. 6 hours
   b. 12 hours
   c. 24 hours
   d. 48 hours

6. How long after transplantation does the kidney reach maximal size?
   a. 12 months
   b. 6 months
   c. 4 months
   d. 2 months

7. Which of the following sonographic images would best demonstrate the presence of a urinoma?
   a. Transverse superior to the kidney
   b. Sagittal at mid-kidney
   c. Transverse bladder
   d. Oblique view of lower pole of kidney and bladder

8. What is normal arterial RI in a transplanted kidney?
   a. 0.5
   b. 0.7
   c. 0.9
   d. 1.0

9. Which velocity is critical to accurately calculate the RI?
   a. Early diastolic
   b. Mid-diastolic
   c. End diastolic
   d. Systolic

10. What pattern of color display in the interlobar arteries is consistent with normal flow?
    a. Flow with minimal diminishment at end diastole
    b. Lack of flow at end diastole
    c. Flashy and pulsatile
    d. Minimal flow at end diastole

11. When does graft loss due to rejection occur?
    a. 3 months
    b. 6 months
    c. 9 months
    d. 12 months

12. What is the medical term for sudden cessation of urine production?
    a. Anuria
    b. Oliguria
    c. Polyuria
    d. Hematuria

13. Which of the following is NOT a risk factor for development of ATN?
    a. Ischemic time
    b. Hypertension
    c. Donor illness
    d. Nonheart beating surgery

14. Which of the following best describes a perinephric collection fluid collection with multiple thin septations?
    a. Hematoma
    b. Urinoma
    c. Hydronephrosis
    d. Lymphocele

15. Which of the following best describes sonographic duplex findings consistent with renal artery thrombosis (RAT)?
    a. Anechoic lumen with low-resistance flow pattern
    b. Anechoic lumen with high-resistance flow pattern
    c. Intraluminal echoes with low-resistance flow pattern
    d. Intraluminal echoes with absence of flow

16. Enlargement of the kidney with decreased renal cortical echogenicity is most consistent with which of the following transplant complications?
    a. Renal artery thrombosis
    b. Renal vein thrombosis
    c. Renal artery stenosis
    d. Lymphocele

17. What is the most common vascular complication following renal transplantation?
    a. Renal artery thrombus
    b. Renal vein thrombus
    c. Renal artery stenosis
    d. Renal artery kink

18. What do Doppler criteria consistent with RAS of >50% to 60% in transplanted kidney include?
    a. PSV >250 cm/s
    b. PSV ratio ≤2.0 to 3.0
    c. AT <70 to 80 ms
    d. Lack of end-diastolic flow

19. Which of the following is NOT a Doppler characteristic of a AVF?
    a. Area of color aliasing
    b. Soft tissue color bruit
    c. High velocity in both systole and diastole
    d. Low velocity in systole and diastole

20. In liver transplants, the arterial anastomosis of hepatic artery is performed by which type of anastomosis?
    a. End to end
    b. Side to side
    c. Fish mouth
    d. Piggy back

21. Which of the following is the most common cause of liver transplant loss?
    a. Rejection
    b. Biliary complication
    c. Surgical technique
    d. Vascular cause

22. Which of the following is NOT a contraindication for liver transplantation?
    a. Renal malignancy
    b. Untreated infection
    c. Hemochromatosis
    d. CHF and COPD

23. The preferred anastomosis of donor CBD is to recipient's:
    a. Common hepatic duct
    b. Common bile duct
    c. Duodenum
    D. Jejunum

24. What is the best patient "window" for sonographic duplex assessment of hepatic transplant?
    a. Infracostal
    b. Midline
    c. Subcostal
    D. Intercostal

25. What is the most common vascular complication of liver transplantation?
    a. Hepatic artery thrombosis
    b. Hepatic artery stenosis
    c. Hepatic artery pseudoaneurysm
    d. Portal vein thrombosis

FILL-IN-THE-BLANK

1. Organs for transplantations are from either
   a _____ donor (DD) or
   _____ donor (LRD).

2. The common causes of end-stage renal disease include:
   _____ _____,
   autosomal _____
   _____ kidney disease,
   glomerulonephritis, _____,
   atherosclerosis, and systemic _____
   _____.

3. Symptoms of renal graft failure might include: _____ , rising _____ level, pain, _____ and fever.

4. The oval piece of donor's aortic wall that contains the main renal artery is called a _____ _____.

5. The donor renal artery is directly anastomosed to the recipient _____ with an end-to-side approach; whereas the donor renal vein is anastomosed to the recipient _____ in an end-to-side approach.

6. The formula to calculate a renal RI is (peak _____ velocity-end- _____ velocity)/ _____ systolic velocity.

7. The types of graft failure that are best managed medically include acute _____ necrosis, _____, _____, and drug _____.

8. Mild _____ is a normal finding postrenal transplantation.

9. Risk factors for renal artery thrombosis include _____ states, _____, intraoperative _____, _____ of vessel size, and vascular _____.

10. The presenting symptom of a patient with renal artery stenosis after a renal transplant is severe _____ _____.

11. The _____ has become the second most common organ to be transplanted after the _____.

12. Liver transplantation is the only available option for patients with acute or chronic _____-stage liver _____ who are unresponsive to _____ therapy.

13. Criteria used to rank patients for liver transplant are _____ and _____ score.

14. If a patient has a _____, bile will drain directly into the _____.

15. In single-lobe LRD transplant, the right portion of the liver will include the right _____ vein, a right _____ vein, a right hepatic _____, and the right hepatic _____ duct.

16. In liver transplantation, hepatic artery stenosis or occlusion is often associated with _____ _____ pathology due to sole blood supply.

17. Liver transplantation involves anastomosis of the _____ system, _____ veins, _____ artery, and _____ duct.

18. Clinical symptoms of hepatic artery stenosis include poor _____ _____ tests or biliary _____.

19. The Doppler waveform in a hepatic artery pseudoaneurysm is _____, showing a typical mix of _____ and _____ signals.

20. When evaluating for possible portal vein thrombosis, the sonographer should use _____ _____ because of the low velocity or absence of flow.

SHORT ANSWER

1. Describe why cadaveric donor allografts continue to be more successful as a transplant option.

2. Explain the methods utilized by the Organ Procurement and Transplantation Network to overcome organ shortage.

3. Describe a typical sonographic protocol for imaging a renal transplant.

4. List at least five causes of true hydronephrosis in a transplanted kidney.

5. List essential components of a liver transplant vascular duplex examination and findings consistent with normal findings.

IMAGE EVALUATION/PATHOLOGY

Review the images and answer the following questions.

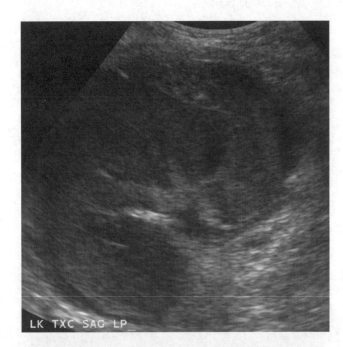

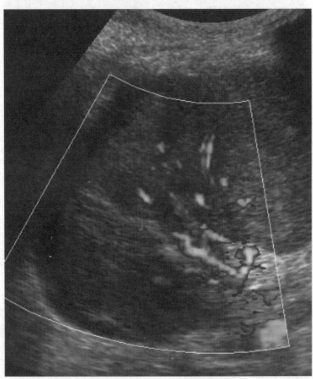

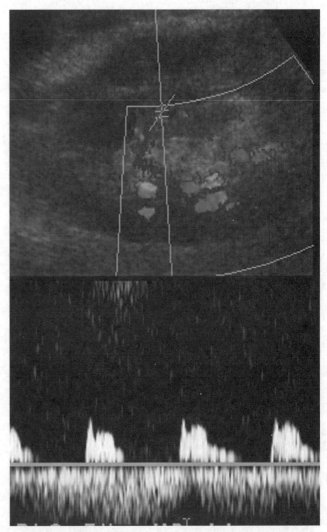

1. These images were taken from the same patient shortly after renal transplant. What is demonstrated in these images?

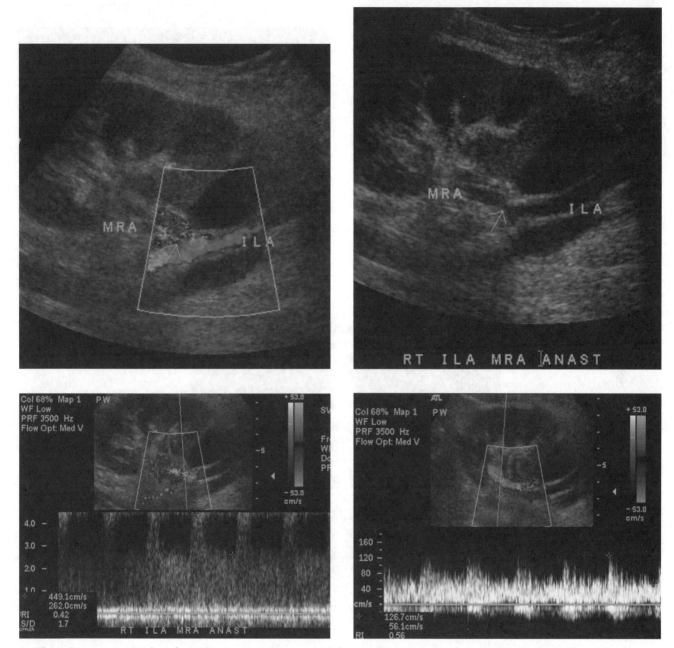

2. These images were taken from the same patient several days postoperatively after renal transplant. The patient presents with severe uncontrolled hypertension. What are these images consistent with?

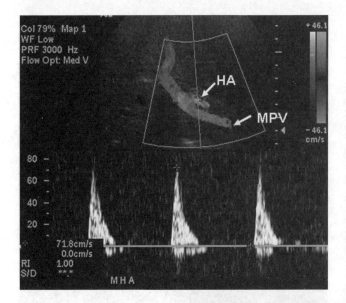

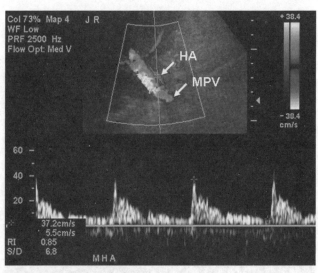

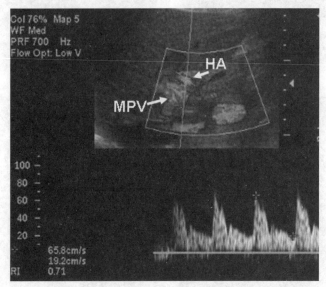

3. This series of images was taken in the main hepatic artery after liver transplant. The first image is immediately postoperative, the next image is 2 days postoperative and the last image is 4 days postoperative. What do these images demonstrate?

CASE STUDY

Review the information and answer the following questions.

1. A 35-year-old female patient who is approximately 3 months post-DD renal transplant presents to the emergency department with oliguria. The lab tests confirm increase in serum creatinine and blood urea nitrogen. She is sent to the ultrasound department for evaluation. As the sonographer, what would you expect to find sonographically and what is the most likely cause for these symptoms?

2. A 57-year-old male patient with a past history of early stage hepatocellular carcinoma treated with a single lobe LRD 3 weeks ago presents for follow-up complaining of nausea and vomiting with increasing jaundice. After drawing LFTs, the patient is sent to the ultrasound lab for evaluation. What types of vascular and nonvascular complications could cause the patient's symptoms?

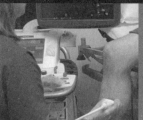

24 Intraoperative Duplex Sonography

REVIEW OF GLOSSARY TERMS

MATCHING

Match the key terms with their definitions.

Key Terms

1. _____ Autologous

2. _____ Endarterectomy

3. _____ Infrainguinal

4. _____ Prosthetic

5. _____ Revascularization

6. _____ Sterile technique

Definition

a. Below the inguinal level; procedure performed below the groin

b. Restoration of blood flow to an organ or area by way of bypass, endarterectomy, or angioplasty and stenting

c. Removal of plaque, intimae, and part of media of an artery to restore normal flow through the diseased segment

d. Means by which a surgical field is isolated from nonsterile or contaminated materials

e. Self-produced or from the same organisms

f. A device replacing an absent or damaged part

CHAPTER REVIEW

MULTIPLE CHOICE

Complete each question by circling the best answer.

1. Which of the following is considered the "gold standard" for intraoperative assessment of any type of revascularization?
   a. Duplex ultrasound
   b. Arteriography
   c. CW Doppler only
   d. Palpation

2. Which duplex ultrasound system requirements would be best suited for intraoperative assessment?
   a. Portable systems with high-frequency transducers
   b. High-end systems with large-array transducers
   c. Grayscale-only systems with high-frequency transducers
   d. Large systems with a variety of transducers

3. What is the primary role of the vascular technologist during intraoperative procedures?
   a. Manipulation of the transducer in the sterile field as well as system operation
   b. Manipulation of the transducer in the sterile field only
   c. Operation of the ultrasound system as the vascular surgeon manipulates the transducer
   d. The vascular technologist does not participate during intraoperative procedures

4. In general, when performing an intraoperative assessment, which of the following imaging techniques is best?
   a. Grayscale imaging only
   b. Spectral Doppler analysis only
   c. Combination of grayscale, color, and spectral Doppler
   d. Color Doppler assessment only

5. What is a benefit of angiography in the intraoperative assessment of carotid endarterectomy?
   a. Ability to visualize the intracranial carotid artery
   b. Ability to visualize the extracranial internal carotid artery
   c. The use of contrast is not needed
   d. It offers physiologic data as well as anatomic data

6. During intraoperative assessment of carotid endarterectomy, spectral Doppler demonstrated velocities of 200 cm/s in the internal carotid artery, while velocities in the common carotid artery were 70 cm/s. Based on these findings, which of the following is likely to occur?
   a. Closure of the surgical site with no further investigation
   b. Closure of the surgical site with duplex assessment performed 1 day postoperatively
   c. Repeat intraoperative duplex assessment 30 minutes later
   d. Revision of the surgical site with repeat duplex assessment after revision

7. Which of the following duplex ultrasound findings is NOT associated with platelet aggregation?
   a. Hypochoic or anechoic material adjacent to vessel wall
   b. Focal elevation in peak systolic velocities
   c. Increased velocity ratios
   d. Linear object visualized parallel to vessel walls

8. Upon duplex assessment of a carotid endarterectomy site, shadowing is noted in the proximal internal carotid artery. What is the most likely cause of this shadowing?
   a. Residual atherosclerotic plaquing at the carotid bulb
   b. Artifact from the prosthetic patch at the endarterectomy site
   c. Occlusion of the internal carotid artery from neointimal hyperplasia
   d. Gain setting too low on the ultrasound system

9. Which of the following can lead to complications or failure of an infrainguinal bypass graft?
   a. Inadequate arterial inflow
   b. Use of prosthetic material below the knee
   c. Significant disease in the outflow vessels
   d. All of the above

10. Which of the following is a main advantage of intraoperative duplex assessment of infrainguinal bypass grafts?
    a. Complete anatomic evaluation of the graft
    b. Identification of retained valves
    c. Physiologic information is gathered as well as anatomic
    d. Shadowing due to prosthetic material will enhance the image

11. What is the preferred bypass conduit for infrainguinal revascularization?
    a. Dacron material
    b. PTFE material
    c. Autologous material
    d. All materials are equally preferred

12. What may abnormally low graft velocities in an infrainguinal bypass graft indicate ?
    a. Poor inflow vessels
    b. Poor outflow vessels
    c. Proximal anastomosis attachment failure
    d. Arteriovenous fistulae

13. Which of the following criteria is used most often when assessing whether to revise an infrainguinal bypass graft during intraoperative assessment?
    a. PSV >180 cm/s and velocity ratio >2.5
    b. PWV <150 cm/s and velocity ratio <1.0
    c. PSV >125 cm/s and velocity ratio >4.0
    d. PSV >250 cm/s and velocity ratio >2.5

14. During intraoperative duplex assessment of a lower extremity bypass graft, turbulent flow is noted in the mid-thigh with elevated diastolic flow noted in the proximal thigh. These findings are consistent with which of the following?
    a. Dissection
    b. Shelf lesion
    c. Intimal flap
    d. Arteriovenous fistula

15. Why may intraoperative duplex ultrasound evaluation of renal artery bypass be preferred over angiography?
    a. Failure of renal artery bypass frequently results in death
    b. Duplex ultrasound avoids the use of contrast in a renal compromised patient
    c. It has been shown to be more accurate than angiography
    d. It does not require the presence of a technologist to operate the equipment

FILL-IN-THE-BLANK

1. Vascular reconstructions that lend themselves to intraoperative application of duplex scanning include carotid _____, _____ bypass, and _____ bypass.

2. A typical transducer used during an intraoperative procedure would be a _____ frequency, "_____ stick" linear array.

3. During an intraoperative procedure, a sterile _____ is placed over the transducer once filled with sterile gel and _____ are removed to reduce interference.

4. In duplex assessment of infrainguinal revascularization, injection of _____ into the bypass is helpful in minimizing the effects of _____.

5. Because prosthetic materials absorb _____, intraoperative scanning of these materials is virtually _____; however, prosthetic _____ in _____ endarterectomy can usually be worked around.

6. Carotid endarterectomy is one of the most _____ operations performed by vascular surgeons and typically has stroke rates below _____%; however, there remains some value of intraoperative assessment in order to minimize residual _____.

7. _____-wave Doppler is probably the most commonly used assessment during carotid endarterectomy; however, _____ -wave Doppler or _____ scanning are being shown to be effective for intraoperative assessment.

8. During duplex assessment of carotid endarterectomy, velocities are obtained from the _____, _____, and _____ carotid arteries, and B-mode images are closely examined for wall _____.

9. Plaque remaining in the proximal

_____ carotid artery

or distal _____ carotid

artery after endarterectomy, which appears

as an abrupt _____ or

_____, is often referred to as a

_____ lesion.

10. An _____ flow is another

complication of endarterectomy and is often revised

if in excess of _____ mm. A less

common complication is _____ as

a result of clamp injury.

11. Infrainguinal revascularization can be perfumed

for _____ or critical

_____ _____.

12. Issues associated with infrainguinal revascularization

include assessing and obtaining adequate arterial

_____, choice of an appropriate

_____, and choice of adequacy of

an _____ target.

13. Methods of assessing bypasses in the operating room

include _____,

_____-wave Doppler,

_____, angioscopy, and

_____ ultrasound scanning.

14. Duplex scanning during lower extremity bypass

allows the entire length of the bypass to be evaluated

to identify retained _____,

_____ areas, arteriovenous

_____ or platelet

_____.

15. Findings that prompt revision of lower extremity

bypass grafts include a peak systolic velocity greater

than _____ cm/s and a velocity

ratio greater than _____.

16. Aortoiliac reconstruction involves

_____ vessels when compared

to carotid or lower extremity procedures, as such

assessment is usually by _____ or

continuous-wave _____.

17. Duplex sonography has distinct advantages

over angiography in the assessment of visceral

revascularizations, including the ability to visualize

small _____ and the lack of the

need for _____, particular for

patients with poor renal function.

18. In renal bypass assessment, velocities of

_____ cm/s by duplex scanning

were an indication for _____.

19. Abnormal intraoperative duplex studies of

mesenteric bypass grafts have been associated with

early _____, graft

_____, and

_____.

20. Criteria for normal results of a mesenteric bypass

graft include peak systolic velocities below

_____ cm/s for the celiac

artery and _____ cm/s for the

superior mesenteric artery, a velocity ratio less

than _____ and no technical

_____.

SHORT ANSWER

1. Describe the preparation that is necessary for both the surgical site and the ultrasound system when used in the operating room. What is the role of the vascular technologist?

2. Compare and contrast the advantages and drawbacks of angiography versus duplex scanning in the intraoperative environment.

IMAGE EVALUATION/PATHOLOGY

Review the images and answer the following questions.

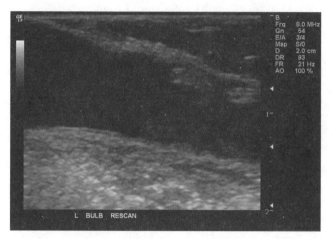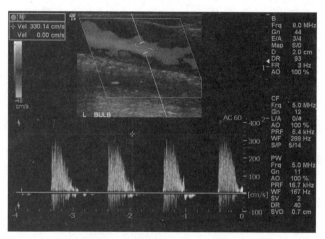

1. You are assisting a vascular surgeon during carotid endarterectomy. During the procedure, the preceding images were obtained.

   a. Describe the findings in these images.

   b. Based on these findings, what would the next course of action likely be?

CASE STUDY

Review the information and answer the following questions.

1. A 65-year-old male is undergoing infrainguinal bypass grafting on the left leg. The vascular surgeon is using autologous veins for the bypass. What specific complications should you be concerned about during the intraoperative evaluation? What findings would likely warrant reexamination and/or revision of the graft?

2. During intraoperative duplex assessment of a superior mesenteric bypass graft, velocities near the distal anastomosis were observed to reach 350 cm/s. What are these findings consistent with? What might the consequences of these findings be?

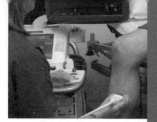

25 The Role of Ultrasound in Central Vascular Access Device Placement

REVIEW OF GLOSSARY TERMS

MATCHING

Match the key terms with their definitions.

Key Terms

1. _____ Air embolism

2. _____ Fistula

3. _____ Guidewire

4. _____ Infiltration

5. _____ Microintroducer

6. _____ PICC

7. _____ Pneumothorax

8. _____ Sheath

9. _____ Stenosis

10. _____ Peel-away sheath

Definition

a. A sheath that is perforated along the long axis, allowing device to be split for removal from a catheter

b. A nitinol or stainless steel wire used to support sheath or catheter exchanges and to predict vessel patency

c. Small needles and wires used to make the initial access into a target

d. Narrowing of a vein or artery due to disease or trauma

e. Collection of air in the pleural space (between lung and chest wall)

f. An abnormal connection or passageway between two organs or vessels, may be created due to trauma or intentionally for therapeutic purposes

g. A thin-walled, hollow plastic tube through which wires and catheters can be advanced

h. Inadvertent release of air or gas into the venous system

i. A peripherally inserted central catheter; a type of vascular access device that is typically inserted into a vein of the upper extremity and threaded to achieve a tip location in the distal third of the superior vena cava

j. Leaking of IV fluid from a catheter into the tissue surrounding the vein

ANATOMY AND PHYSIOLOGY REVIEW

IMAGE LABELING

Complete the labels in the images that follow.

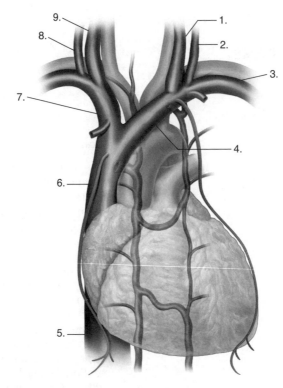

The central veins.

CHAPTER REVIEW

MULTIPLE CHOICE

Complete each question by circling the best answer.

1. Central venous access may be used in patients requiring which of the following?
   a. Intravenous antibiotic therapy
   b. Chemotherapy
   c. Total parenteral nutrition
   d. All of the above

2. Which of the following is NOT one of the most commonly used peripheral access points for VAD placement?
   a. Basilic vein
   b. Cephalic vein
   c. Popliteal vein
   d. Internal jugular vein

3. Why is the atriocaval junction a desirable location for placement of the VAD catheter tip?
   a. Flow rates are around 2,000 mL/min
   b. Blood flows directly into the left atrium from this location
   c. Flow rates are typically lower for better dispersion
   d. The atriocaval junction is NOT a desirable location

4. What is a type of VAD that is placed percutaneously into a central or peripheral vein within its end secured at the puncture site known as?
   a. Tunneled central VAD
   b. Nontunneled central VAD
   c. Implanted port
   d. Port-a-cath

5. Which of the following is a type of VAD in which the catheter exits the skin away from the puncture site?
   a. Tunneled central VAD
   b. Nontunneled central VAD
   c. Implanted port
   d. Port-a-cath

6. Which of the following is NOT a benefit of a tunneled central VAD?
   a. Reduction of device-related infection
   b. More stable device
   c. Hidden exit site for cosmetic reasons
   d. Less comfortable for the patient

7. Implanted ports are typically used in patients who require therapy at what rate?
   a. Daily
   b. Weekly
   c. Every few hours
   d. Continuously

8. Which of the following veins is typically the first choice for placement of peripherally inserted central catheters (PICCs)?
   a. Cephalic
   b. Brachial
   c. Basilic
   d. Axillary

9. For which of the following patients would it be more common to use the saphenous vein for central vascular access placement?
   a. 75-year-old woman
   b. 2-day-old infant
   c. 35-year-old male
   d. 62-year-old male

10. Which of the following describes the preferred use of peripheral cannulas?
    a. Long-term (more than 1 year), continuous therapy
    b. Long-term, intermittent therapy
    c. Therapy lasting several months
    d. Short-term therapy (less than 1 week)

11. Which jugular vein is preferred for central VAD placement?
    a. Right internal jugular vein
    b. Left internal jugular vein
    c. Right external jugular vein
    d. Left external jugular vein

12. Where is the internal jugular vein typically located in relation to the common carotid artery?
    a. Directly lateral
    b. Directly anterior
    c. Anterolateral
    d. Anteromedial

13. Because of their location around the clavicle, which of the following vessels is more difficult to visualize with ultrasound?
    a. Axillary vein
    b. Subclavian vein
    c. Internal jugular vein
    d. Basilic vein

14. Which of the following is a reason to avoid use of the common femoral vein in VAD placement?
    a. Difficult to visualize on ultrasound
    b. Preservation for use for lower extremity bypass grafting
    c. Low flow rates
    d. Higher rate of mechanical and infectious complications

15. Which of the following is NOT included in the initial assessment for potential access sites for VAD placement?
    a. Patency of the vessel
    b. Location of vessel in relation to other structures
    c. Blood flow velocity
    d. Ability to access the target vessel

16. How is confirmation of tip placement of a vascular access device typically made?
    a. Ultrasound
    b. Chest x-ray
    c. CT scan
    d. Contrast MRA

17. A patient presents to the vascular lab after VAD placement to evaluate the basilic vein in which the device is placed. Upon ultrasound evaluation, the basilic vein is noted to have an irregular intimal surface with low-level echoes within the vein lumen. What are these findings consistent with?
    a. Nontarget puncture and hematoma
    b. Air embolism in the basilic vein
    c. Vein damage with thrombosis
    d. Arteriovenous fistula

18. Which of the following is one of the most serious and potentially life-threatening complications of central venous catheterization?
    a. Pneumothorax
    b. Arteriovenous fistula
    c. Thrombosis
    d. Vein wall damage

19. Which of the following medications would be associated with an increased risk of bleeding during vascular access device placement?
    a. Clopidrogel
    b. Warfarin
    c. Heparin
    d. All of the above

20. Which of the following complications of VAD placement is often transient and results in few, if any, symptoms?
    a. Vein wall damage
    b. Cardiac arrhythmias
    c. Arteriovenous fistula
    d. Pneumothorax

FILL-IN-THE-BLANK

1. When matching vascular access devices to that patient, one must consider therapy _____, number and type of _____, and patient _____ and activity _____.

2. The most common target veins for central vascular access devices include the _____ and _____ veins in the medial arm, the _____ vein in the lateral arm, and the more centrally located _____ and internal _____ veins.

3. The catheter tip of a vascular access device typically resides in the _____ third of the _____ _____ _____ at the _____ junction.

4. Nontunneled access devices are typically used for patients requiring access for _____ to _____ , whereas tunneled vascular access devices can remain in place for _____.

5. Implanted _____ are vascular access devices with a _____ segment attached to a plastic or titanium _____.

6. Because of the location of the brachial veins next to the _____ artery, there is a higher risk of inadvertent arterial _____ if the brachial veins are used for peripheral VAD placement.

7. The most common sites for central venous access are the internal _____ vein and the _____ veins.

8. Ultrasound allows for _____ assessment of the internal jugular vein prior to VAD placement as well as dynamic _____ during vein puncture.

9. Using ultrasound guidance during vein puncture can reduce _____ of catheter placement as well as complication rates related to _____.

10. When using ultrasound guidance, it is important to assess the _____ of the vessel, vessel _____, vessel _____, and variations in diameter with _____.

11. Neither the _____ nor other upper extremity veins should be used for cannulation in patients with chronic _____ insufficiency or _____ kidney disease in order to preserve these vessels for _____ in the future.

12. The common femoral veins are most often sued for central venous access in _____ situations and in patients in whom other potential access veins are _____.

13. Patency of a vessel for potential access is first tested by _____, similar to that used in the assessment of a patient for deep venous _____.

14. Under ultrasound guidance, the needle used for access should be visualized once it enters the _____, as it approaches the _____ vessel, and as a successful _____ has been attained.

15. Complications associated with central venous access device placement include vein _____, nontarget _____, bleeding, air _____, and cardiac _____.

16. The presence of _____ veins upon physical exam should alert the clinician to potential _____ in successful placement of VADs.

17. Examples of complications due to vein damage include blood _____ and _____ fistula.

18. In order to minimize the impact of non-_____puncture, a small _____ _____ should be used.

19. Bleeding with or following VAD placement may occur due to difficult VAD _____ , _____ disorders, and concurrent treatment with certain _____.

20. The risk of air embolism can be minimized by using _____ sheaths, performing _____ maneuvers efficiently, and assuring that catheter lumens are _____, secured, and _____.

SHORT ANSWER

1. List the types of available vascular access devices and the typical uses of each.

2. Describe the scanning technique and key uses of ultrasound guidance during vascular access device placement.

IMAGE EVALUATION/PATHOLOGY

Review the images and answer the following questions.

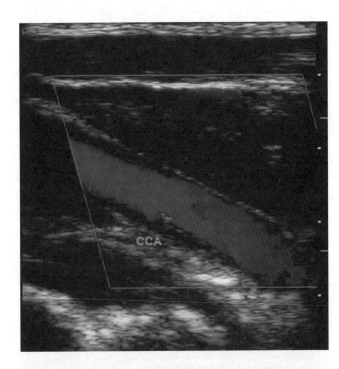

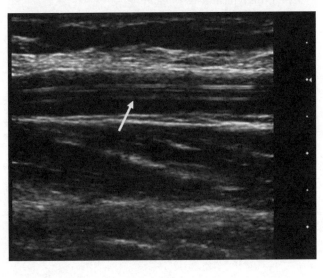

1. This image was taken from the proximal neck. What are these findings consistent with?

2. This image was taken in the mid-medial upper arm. What is shown in this image? Does this appear normal or abnormal?

CASE STUDY

Review the information and answer the following questions.

1. A 63-year-old female presents for evaluation of a central vascular access device that was placed through the internal jugular vein. A pulsatile mass was noted in the patient's neck. With this limited clinical information, what would the most likely cause of the pulsatile mass be and what would be expected on the ultrasound examination?

2. A 57-year-old male presents for ultrasound evaluation after subclavian vein VAD placement. On the ultrasound examination, a hypoechoic area is noted adjacent to the subclavian vein. What are these findings consistent with and what complications may arise?

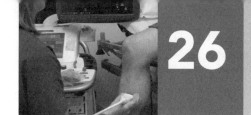

REVIEW OF GLOSSARY TERMS

MATCHING

Match the key terms with their definitions.

Key Terms

1. _____ Hemodialysis access

2. _____ Arteriovenous fistula

3. _____ Arteriovenous graft

Definition

a. An abnormal connection between an artery and vein; may be congenital or acquired

b. A type of hemodialysis access that uses a prosthetic conduit to connect an artery to a vein to allow for dialysis

c. Also known as vascular access, a surgically created connection between an artery and vein to allow for removal of toxic products from the blood by dialysis

ANATOMY AND PHYSIOLOGY REVIEW

IMAGE LABELING

Complete the labels in the images that follow.

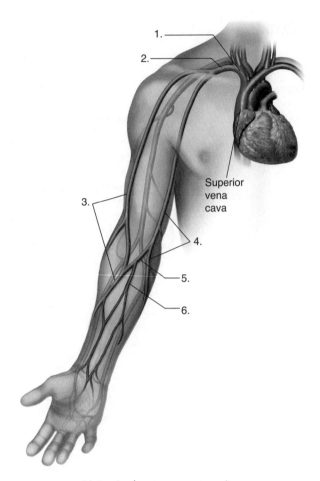

Superior
vena
cava

Veins in the upper extremity.

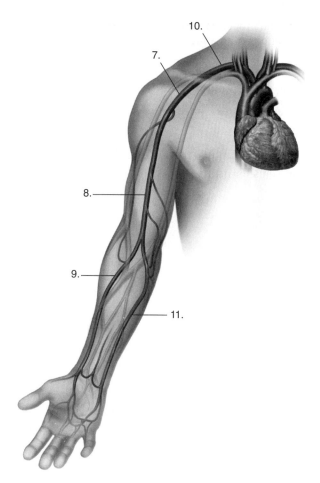

Arteries in the upper extremity.

CHAPTER REVIEW

MULTIPLE CHOICE

Complete each question by circling the best answer.

1. The goal of the Kidney Dialysis Outcomes Quality Initiative and the Fistula First Breakthrough Initiative was to increase and expand the creation of which of the following?
   a. Prosthetic hemodialysis access grafts
   b. Autogenous hemodialysis access fistulae
   c. Lower extremity hemodialysis access
   d. Central venous port access

2. What is maturation failure of dialysis access fistulae most commonly due to?
   a. Small or suboptimal veins
   b. Venous outflow stenosis
   c. Arterial inflow stenosis
   d. Arterial steal syndrome

3. Which of the following should be included during the physical examination for preoperative artery mapping for dialysis fistula creation?
   a. Bilateral arm blood pressure measurements
   b. Pulse exam of brachial, radial, and ulnar arteries
   c. Allen test for palmar arch assessment
   d. All of the above

4. Which of the following is NOT a finding suggestive of a central venous stenosis or occlusion?
   a. Arm edema
   b. Prominent chest wall veins
   c. Painful, cool, pale hand
   d. Presence of arm collaterals

5. Which of the following describes the proper patient positioning for upper extremity venous evaluation prior to fistula creation?
   a. Supine with arm elevated
   b. Supine or sitting with arm dependent
   c. Standing with weight held in arm to be examined
   d. Trendelenburg with feet elevated

6. What does standard protocol for evaluation of the upper extremity arteries and veins for fistula creation begin with?
   a. Veins of dominant arm
   b. Veins of nondominant arm
   c. Arteries of dominant arm
   d. Arteries of nondominant arm

7. What is the acceptable size for upper extremity arteries before fistula creation?
   a. >2.0 mm
   b. >2.5 mm
   c. <3.0 mm
   d. <2.0 mm

8. All Doppler studies should be performed at an angle of _____ or less, even if actual velocities are not recorded in order to achieve adequate Doppler signals.
   a. 75°
   b. 60°
   c. 90°
   d. 0°

9. What is the acceptable minimum vein diameter for favorable fistula creation?
   a. 2.0 mm
   b. 1.5 mm
   c. 2.5 mm
   d. 1.0 mm

10. Which of the following should venous Doppler signals from central veins NOT display?
    a. Respiratory phasicity
    b. Cardiac pulsatility
    c. Augmentation
    d. Continuous flow

11. What is a type of fistula created by connecting the posterior branch of the radial artery to the cephalic vein?
    a. Brescia-Cimino fistula
    b. Transposition fistula
    c. Snuffbox fistula
    d. Berman-Gentile fistula

12. The most common upper arm access is made between the cephalic vein and which artery?
    a. Subclavian artery
    b. Brachial artery
    c. Axillary artery
    d. Brachiocephalic artery

13. Approximately how long should it take an autogenous fistula to mature?
    a. 8 to 12 weeks
    b. 1 to 3 days
    c. 6 to 8 months
    d. 1 to 2 years

14. During evaluation of the upper extremity either before or after fistula creation, the examination should be kept warm to avoid what?
    a. Vasodilation
    b. Vasospasm
    c. The use of coupling gel
    d. Ultrasound equipment failure

15. Which of the following is NOT included in a physical examination of a patient with a current AV fistula?
    a. Assessment of thrill
    b. Assessment for edema or redness
    c. Bilateral radial blood pressures
    d. Visual inspection for focal dilations and collateral veins

16. During duplex assessment of the dialysis fistula, what should Doppler settings be adjusted to detect?
    a. Low flow
    b. Continuous flow
    c. Intermittent flow
    d. High flow

17. Which of the following describes how volumetric flow is calculated?
    a. Time average velocity/PSV
    b. Time average velocity × area × 60
    c. Time average velocity × vessel diameter
    d. PSV − EDV/PSV

18. What can remaining valve leaflets that project into the lumen of a fistula become a source for?
    a. Dissection
    b. Pseudoaneurysm development
    c. Stenosis development
    d. Calcium deposition

19. A patient presents to the vascular lab for follow-up evaluation of a dialysis fistula. Velocities within the fistula are 40 cm/s. What are these findings consistent with?
    a. Normal fistula function
    b. Fistula pseudoaneurysm
    c. Perigraft mass
    d. Inflow artery stenosis

20. Normal volume flow in a fistula should be approximately what?
    a. 200 mL/min
    b. 500 mL/min
    c. 800 mL/min
    d. 100 mL/min

FILL-IN-THE-BLANK

1. The goal of arteriovenous access is to provide _____-_____ hemodialysis access with a _____ frequency of reintervention and a low _____ rate.

2. _____ access has been the preferred first-line therapy because it has superior _____ rates and lower _____ rates compared to _____ grafts.

3. AV fistulas have higher long-term _____ rates; however, they suffer from lower _____ rates and higher early _____ rates.

4. Risk factors that may preclude the creation of an arteriovenous hemodialysis fistula include placement of central venous _____, _____, _____, or prior _____ with lymph node dissection.

5. AV fistula creation is usually first attempted in the non_____ upper extremity as far _____ as possible.

6. When assessing arteries for AV fistula placement, they should be assessed for _____ , _____ thickness, _____, and compliance.

7. When assessing veins for AV fistula placement, B-mode imaging should confirm that the veins walls are _____ and free of _____, webbing, and _____.

8. Contraindications to ultrasound assessment of upper extremity arteries and veins for fistula placement include _____ lines, _____, open _____, and limited patient _____.

9. Maturation of a hemodialysis fistula is defined as a _____, easily _____, usable fistula with a flow rate of _____ cc/min.

10. A partially or non_____ vein suggests the presence of an occluding _____ within the vein lumen, making it _____ as an autogenous conduit.

11. A Brescia-Cimino fistula is the most frequently created fistula and involves the _____ vein and the _____ artery at the _____.

12. Because of its _____ location, the _____ vein requires that it be _____ and juxtaposed to a distal artery in order to create an AV fistula.

13. Fistulae and grafts should be followed up consistently. Indications for follow-up include _____, either in outflow vein or anastomoses; _____ formation; _____ formation; or arterial _____.

14. During physical assessment of a patient with an access fistula, the technologist should visually inspect the arm for _____, _____, presence of _____ veins, rotation of the _____ sites, and focal _____.

15. During B-mode evaluation of a dialysis fistula or graft, it is important to assess for abnormalities including perigraft _____, _____, stenotic _____, and _____ flaps.

16. Doppler evaluation of the fistula or graft includes documentation of _____ of the fistula as well as identifying any areas of _____. When stenosis is found, velocities should be measured _____, _____, and _____ the area of interest.

17. _____ flow measurements are useful when evaluating access function. Use of the _____ average velocity is used in this measurement and is best measured over _____ to _____ cardiac cycles to obtain an accurate calculation.

18. Abnormal findings within a fistula include bright white reflectors in the walls consistent with _____, _____, either hypoechoic or anechoic; _____ leaflets projecting into the vessel lumen; and elevated velocities consistent with _____.

19. Normal findings in a well-functioning fistula include PSV between _____ and _____ cm/s with EDV of _____ cm/s, marked _____ broadening, and continuous _____ diastolic flow.

20. _____ and _____ stenoses account for the majority of access complications. Stenosis in fistula evaluation is indicated when PSV increases by _____% or a velocity ratio of _____.

SHORT ANSWER

1. Why is it important for the inflow artery to a dialysis access fistula to be free of calcifications and/or atherosclerosis?

2. When would it be appropriate to use the lower extremity for fistula creation? What vessels can be used?

3. List the indications for fistula assessment after it has been placed.

4. Describe the symptoms and sonographic findings associated with arterial steal syndrome.

5. Describe the sonographic findings in a normal hemodialysis fistula, including arterial inflow within the fistula and outflow vein.

IMAGE EVALUATION/PATHOLOGY

Review the images and answer the following questions.

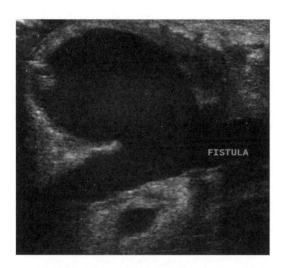

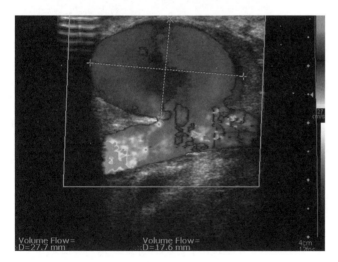

1. The images shown on the left were taken from the mid-forearm. What is demonstrated?

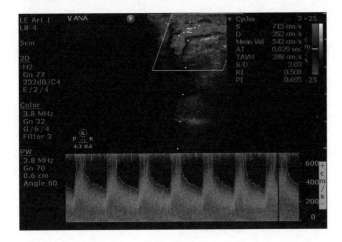

2. This image demonstrates that anastomosis of a dialysis access fistula. What is demonstrated here?

CASE STUDY

Review the information and answer the following questions.

1. A right-handed patient presents to the vascular laboratory for upper extremity evaluation prior to hemodialysis access creation. What protocol would you use to evaluate this patient and what criteria would you use to determine if the vessels are adequate for fistula placement?

2. A patient presents to the vascular lab with elevated venous pressure during dialysis. What findings would you expect on your duplex assessment of this fistula?

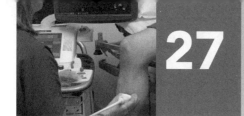

27 Vascular Applications of Ultrasound Contrast Agents

REVIEW OF GLOSSARY TERMS

MATCHING

Match the key terms with their definitions.

Key Terms

1. _____ Ultrasound contrast agent

2. _____ Microbubbles

3. _____ Contrast-enhanced sonography

Definition

a. The use of medical ultrasound imaging after administration of an ultrasound contrast agent

b. Compositions that, after administration, alter the acoustic properties of body tissues, typically resulting in higher ultrasound signal reflectivity

c. Encapsulated gas-containing structures that are typically smaller than 8 microns in size

CHAPTER REVIEW

MULTIPLE CHOICE

Complete each question by circling the best answer.

1. The "bubbles" used for ultrasound contrast are typically smaller than what?
   a. 2 microns
   b. 4 microns
   c. 6 microns
   d. 8 microns

2. Contrast agents are approved for use in the United States for which of the following?
   a. Abdominal organ
   b. Echocardiography
   c. Peripheral vascular
   d. Retroperitoneal

3. Which of the following is NOT a disadvantage of using saline as a contrast agent?
   a. Persist through pulmonary circulation
   b. Nonuniform in size
   c. Relatively large size
   d. Unstable or fragile

4. What is the microbubble shell in Definity?
   a. Human serum albumin
   b. Lipid
   c. Galactose and palmitic acid
   d. Phospholipid

5. Which of the following is NOT a characteristic of a viable contrast agent?
   a. Nontoxic to a wide variety of patients
   b. Microparticles that pass pulmonary capillary bed
   c. Size greater than 8 microns
   d. Stable to recirculate through CV system

6. How is the ultrasound contrast agent administered?
   a. Oral
   b. Intramuscular
   c. Intravenous
   d. Central line

7. Approximately how long will contrast administered in a bolus dose provide enhanced visualization?
   a. 2 min
   b. 4 min
   c. 8 min
   d. 12 min

8. Which of the following applications would be best suited for slow IV infusion of contrast agent?
   a. Cardiac chamber opacification
   b. Identification of large vessel wall
   c. Identification of aneurysm
   d. Organ perfusion

9. After the microbubbles are ruptured, how are the shell particles removed from the body?
   a. Metabolized
   b. Absorption
   c. Excretion
   d. Exhalation

10. Which type of UCA would best serve a patient/ sonographer when the diagnosis is DVT and vessels are difficult to visualize?
    a. Blood pool agent
    b. Molecular imaging agent
    c. Thrombus-specific agent
    d. Tissue-specific agent

11. Which of the following is NOT an ultrasound system setting necessary for successful use of contrast agents?
    a. Flash echo
    b. Low mechanical index
    c. High acoustic output power
    d. Harmonic imaging

12. Which of the following situations would most likely be enhanced with the use of contrast ultrasound agent?
    a. Carotid with diagnostic level images
    b. Deep vessels with luminal echogenicity
    c. Vessels with slow flow identified by power Doppler
    d. Postoperative complicated bypass surgery

13. In PAD, in which situation would using contrast agent improve the diagnostic quality of examination?
    a. Atherosclerotic plaque on posterior vessel wall
    b. Occlusion of the proximal femoral artery
    c. Perfusion deficit of calf muscle
    d. DVT of popliteal vein

14. Which of the following does NOT limit sonographic visualization of intracranial vessels?
    a. Acoustic windows
    b. High-velocity flow
    c. Signal attenuation
    d. Vessel branches

15. In which situation is duplex sonography least effective in the evaluation of organ transplant?
    a. Postsurgical fluid collections
    b. Urinary or bile obstructions
    c. Blood flow to and from organ
    d. Tissue perfusion

16. What is the most significant advantage to CES over repeated CT for evaluation of endovascular leaks?
    a. Real-time blood flow assessment
    b. Lack of ionizing radiation
    c. Less chance of renal failure
    d. Ability to detect leak flow

17. What would the use of contrast-enhanced ultrasound in the abdominal vasculature prove MOST helpful in?
    a. Renal artery stent demonstrating laminar flow
    b. Abdominal aortic aneurysm demonstrating true and false lumen
    c. Turbulent blood flow through a TIPS
    d. Competent endovascular graft of abdominal aorta

18. In a cardiac application, what would the use of a saline contrast study help diagnose?
    a. Left-to-right shunting VSD
    b. Patent ductus arteriosus
    c. Left ventricular aneurysm
    d. Patent foramen ovale

19. When assessing for vessel occlusion with contrast-enhanced sonography, what are the expected findings?
    a. Vessel visualization distal to occlusion
    b. Vessel visualization with no enhanced distal flow
    c. Delayed vessel opacification
    d. Visualization of flow "around" echogenic plaque in vessel

20. What would contrast-enhanced sonographic imaging in the cerebrovascular circulation prove helpful in?
    a. Delineation of plaque ulceration
    b. Assessment of functional lumen
    c. Identification of string flow
    d. All of the above

FILL-IN-THE-BLANK

1. Ultrasound contrast agents alter the

   _____ _____

   of body tissues, resulting in _____

   signal reflectivity.

2. The use of contrast agents has been shown to

   _____ or _____

   limitations of ultrasound imaging, which include

   _____ _____

   on grayscale, _____ blood flow,

   and small _____.

3. When a vascular agent's microbubbles are ruptured or otherwise destroyed, the shell products

   are _____ and the gas is

   _____.

4. Tissue-specific agents must possess two unique

   characteristics: _____ for the

   targeted tissue and ability to alter that tissue's

   _____ appearance.

5. Tissue-specific UCAs target specific types of tissues

   with a predictable behavior, so they are considered

   _____ _____

   _____.

6. Although blood-pool agents help to better delineate

   the functional _____ of arteries

   and veins, they do not enhance the appearance of

   _____.

7. Thrombus-targeting UCAs have a

   _____ function by enhancing

   _____ when insonated.

8. _____ imaging is performed

   with the same transducers as used for conventional

   ultrasound. The _____

   _____ frequency is

   _____ the transmit frequency.

9. In harmonic imaging, the echoes from
   _____ microbubbles have
   a _____ signal to noise
   _____ than conventional
   ultrasound imaging.

10. When contrast _____ are
    destroyed in an organ, the sonographer is able to
    observe _____ of the tissue.

11. Echocardiography is the most common
    application of UCAs. This application allows
    for improved _____ of
    _____ borders, assessment
    of regional _____
    _____, and detection of
    intracavitary _____.

12. Some of the main limitations in iliac vessel
    visualization are overlying _____
    _____ and
    _____ vessels.

13. In peripheral artery disease evaluations of
    symptomatic patients, the two areas of improved
    visualization with CSE are _____
    _____ and
    _____ _____.

14. Contrast agents are most frequently administered
    via _____ extremity
    _____ access site.

15. The use of contrast-enhanced sonography in
    the cerebrovascular circulation can be used
    to differentiate _____
    _____ from
    _____.

16. Some investigators have compared
    _____ _____
    to tumors because of the requirement of nutrient-rich
    _____ _____
    to grow.

17. Abdominal vascular applications of contrast-
    enhanced imaging include _____
    and its branches, systemic _____,
    _____ venous system, and
    abdominal _____.

18. A significant number of patients have
    anatomical variations of renal vasculature,
    including _____ or
    _____ renal arteries.

19. Identification of abdominal vascular pathology
    that might be enhanced by contrast sonography
    includes _____ ischemia, aortic
    _____, _____
    or _____, and IVC filter
    _____.

20. Contrast agents available for use in the
    United States are _____
    and _____. Unfortunately,
    _____ is the only FDA-approved
    application for contrast agents.

SHORT ANSWER

1. Describe clinical situations where using a bolus
   injection would be more beneficial than slow IV
   infusion.

2. List at least three different types of contrast agents.

IMAGE EVALUATION/PATHOLOGY

Review the images and answer the following questions.

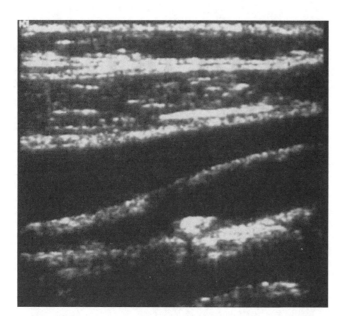

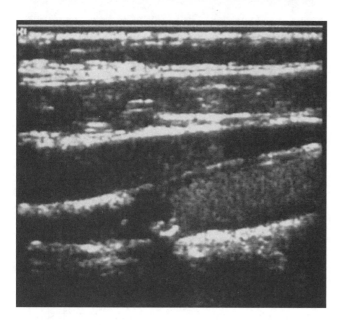

1. These images were taken from the mid-neck near the carotid bulb. What is demonstrated in these images? Is this clear from just the grayscale image?

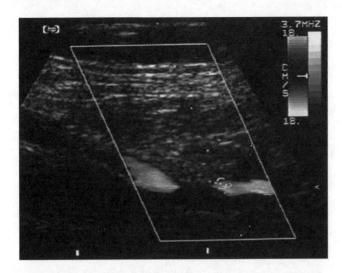

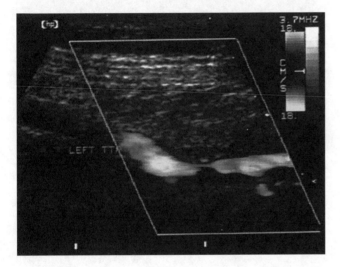

2. These images were obtained through the mid-calf. Describe the findings before and after contrast injection.

CASE STUDY

Review the information and answer the following questions.

1. A 67-year-old male patient with known peripheral vascular disease presents to the emergency department complaining of acute onset PAD symptoms in his right lower extremity. The patient was discharged just 3 days ago after undergoing surgical revascularization of the limb with new symptoms. If contrast-enhanced imaging were available, describe the potential sonographic findings in this patient.

2. A 57-year-old female with numerous cardiovascular risk factors presents for a cerebrovascular duplex examination. She has a left carotid bruit and has recently experienced visual disturbances in her right eye and left-sided weakness that have slowly resolved. What might you expect to see with and without the use of contrast-enhanced sonography?

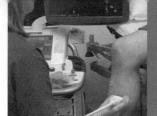
REVIEW OF GLOSSARY TERMS

MATCHING

Match the key terms with their definitions.

Key Terms

1. _____ Gold standard

2. _____ Accuracy

3. _____ Sensitivity

4. _____ Specificity

5. _____ Positive predictive value

6. _____ Negative predictive value

Definition

a. The ability of a test to correctly identify a normal result

b. The proportion of patients with positive test results that are correctly identified

c. The overall percentage of correct results

d. The proportion of negative test results when there is no underlying disease present

e. The ability of a test to detect disease

f. A well-established and reliable testing parameter, which for vascular disease is often angiography

CHAPTER REVIEW

MULTIPLE CHOICE

Complete each question by circling the best answer.

1. In vascular testing, what is typically considered to be the gold standard?
   a. Computed tomography
   b. Magnetic resonance imaging
   c. Angiography
   d. Duplex ultrasound

2. What is the identification of a 50% to 79% stenosis of the internal carotid artery and a 60% stenosis by angiography an example of?
   a. True positive
   b. True negative
   c. False positive
   d. False negative

3. Upon ultrasound evaluation, DVT is found in the popliteal vein; however, venography demonstrates a widely patent vessel. What is this an example of?
   a. True positive
   b. True negative
   c. False positive
   d. False negative

4. During duplex assessment of the abdominal aorta, the aorta measures <2.0 cm, which is confirmed by angiography. What is this an example of?
   a. True positive
   b. True negative
   c. False positive
   d. False negative

5. Duplex evaluation of the superior mesenteric artery demonstrated velocities of 150 cm/s. Angiography demonstrated a 70% stenosis in the same vessel. What is this an example of?
   a. True positive
   b. True negative
   c. False positive
   d. False negative

6. Which of the following is NOT likely to occur if false positive results are indicated by the duplex ultrasound exam?
   a. Unnecessary treatment
   b. Lack of treatment when treatment is needed
   c. Unnecessary stress to the patient
   d. Repeat examinations

7. Which of the following would have the highest accuracy?
   a. 25 true positives and 30 true negatives out of 100 exams
   b. 20 true positives and 10 true negatives out of 100 exams
   c. 50 true positives and 5 true negatives out of 100 exams
   d. 10 true positives and 75 true negatives out of 100 exams

8. An increase in which of the following results would increase the sensitivity of an exam?
   a. False positive
   b. False negative
   c. True positive
   d. True negative

9. Which results are needed to improve specificity?
   a. True negatives
   b. True positives
   c. False negatives
   d. False positives

10. What is the consistency of obtaining similar results under similar circumstances?
    a. Accuracy
    b. Sensitivity
    c. Reliability
    d. Specificity

11. An increase in the number of false positive results would have an impact on which of the following?
    a. Positive predictive value and negative predictive value
    b. Positive predictive value and specificity
    c. Negative predictive value and sensitivity
    d. Positive predictive value and sensitivity

12. After statistical analysis a test was found to have a sensitivity of 92% and a specificity of 84%. Which of the following could represent the overall accuracy?
    a. 95%
    b. 82%
    c. 89%
    d. Cannot be determined

13. If a test has a negative predictive value of 50%, how sure can you be that your test results are negative?
    a. Extremely sure
    b. Moderately sure
    c. Equivocal
    d. Not sure at all

14. In general, if the sensitivity of a test increases, what will happen to the specificity of the test?
    a. Also increase
    b. Decrease
    c. Remain the same
    d. Cannot be determined

15. An increase in the number of false negative results would impact which of the following parameters?
    a. Negative predictive value and sensitivity
    b. Positive predicative value and sensitivity
    c. Sensitivity and specificity
    d. Negative predictive value and specificity

FILL-IN-THE-BLANK

1. Quality _____ refers to a program for the systematic _____ and _____ of the various aspects of vascular testing to ensure that _____ of quality are being met.

2. _____ is the science of making effective use of _____ data relating to groups of individuals or _____.

3. A _____ standard is used to compare one form of a newer _____ test with another that is well _____ and _____.

4. True _____ are the number of studies performed by ultrasound, which state that disease is present and the gold standard _____ with the ultrasound findings.

5. True _____ are the number of studies performed by ultrasound, which state that disease is not present and are also reported as _____ by the gold standard.

6. Studies that are reported positive by ultrasound but are found to be _____ by the gold standard are known as _____ positives.

7. If a study is normal on _____ but the gold standard identifies disease, it is an example of a _____ negative.

8. Accuracy is calculated as the _____ number of correct tests _____ by the total number of all tests.

9. _____ is calculated by taking the _____ positive results and dividing these by all positive results as determined by the _____ _____.

10. Dividing the number of true negatives by all the _____ results as identified by the gold standard results in the _____ of the test.

11. A vascular laboratory that has an overall accuracy of 96% over an average of 5 years would be said to be _____.

12. _____ predictive value is calculated as the number of true _____ divided by all the positive studies.

13. True _____ divided by all studies determined to be negative results in the _____ predictive value.

14. In a chi-square analysis, boxes A and B are

    used to determine _____

    _____ _____,

    whereas boxes C and D are used to determine

    _____ _____

    _____.

15. In a chi-square analysis, boxes A and C are used to

    determine _____,

    whereas boxes B and D are used to determine

    _____.

SHORT ANSWER

1. As the technical director of the vascular laboratory, you are asked to complete a statistical analysis of a particular duplex test. You collect the following data:

    150 test results that were negative both by duplex and angiography

    75 test results that were positive both by duplex and angiography

    15 test results that were positive by duplex but negative by angiography

    10 test results that were negative by duplex but positive by angiography

    What are the sensitivity, specificity, positive predictive value, negative predictive value, and overall accuracy for this test?

2. In examining another test, you collect the following data: 500 total tests of which 300 were negative. Of the negative tests, 200 agreed with the gold standard. Of the positive tests, 100 agreed with the gold standard. What are the sensitivity, specificity, positive predictive value, negative predictive value, and overall accuracy of this test? How would you interpret these results?